D0729293

Macrobiotics for American.
by
Roger Mason

ISBN 1-884820-70-0
Library of Congress Catalog Card #2002106957
Categories: 1. Health 2. Diet

Printed in the U.S.A.
1st Printing August 2002

Published by Safe Goods
561 Shunpike Road
Sheffield, MA 01257
(413) 229-7935

Zen

Macrobiotics

for

Americans

A Practical and Delicious Way to Eat Your Way to Health

Roger Mason

Contents

About This Book

Back in the late sixties most of the middle class youth of America seem to have joined the psychedelic generation and looked for new horizons to expand their lives. Most all of these young people had grown up on meat, potatoes, white bread and sugar as this is all they knew. Along came very conservative George Ohsawa and talked about a way of health and longevity that expanded your mind naturally by being in tune with the universal order. This was appealing to many people and became rather popular along with the general interest in natural food and herbal healing. Now over three decades macrobiotics is still popular and well known.

As I got older and had practiced this way of eating for over thirty years I noticed that all the books were, in fact, on JAPANESE macrobiotics written by Japanese people (or with their outlook) with Japanese cooking. Someone needed to write a book making macrobiotics more PRACTICAL, more down to earth, more fun, tastier, more creative, less restrictive, and just plain more American without watering it down or weakening it at all. There were just too many unneeded limitations and too much cultural influence that simply did not translate here. Foods included expensive, hard to find Japanese vegetables, only allowed 5% of the time, tea with caffeine, buckwheat noodles with white flour, refined couscous, very limited seasonings and condiments, few fresh green and yellow vegetables, with all that salt. There were no supplements or natural hormones, almost no raw foods, sprouts or fresh salads, and did not include fasting

All the books on macrobiotics followed this same Japanese path without deviating. Someone needed to write a book that would keep the integrity and effectiveness of macrobiotics while expanding the scope of it. This will not be a long book, nor filled with recipes and personal stories. At first this may seem like too austere a way to eat everyday, but more and more it becomes your natural way of life and you enjoy it. You no longer want to eat meat, dairy, desserts or tropical foods except very occasionally if at all. After more than 30 years of personally doing this you can believe that this is a wonderful, fulfilling and rewarding way to live as well as the best way to cure "incurable" illnesses.

Overview

There are many natural health books today about the right foods to eat with many contradictory philosophies. How can one know what is valid and what is not? The answer is very simple - RESULTS. The macrobiotic way of eating is the only means I've seen for curing "incurable" illnesses like cancers, diabetes, heart and artery problems, epilepsy and the wide variety of illnesses that plague modern society especially the developed nations.

You have to experience this for yourself. Nature is the greatest healer and our lifestyle allows Nature to heal us. If we are in harmony with the Natural Order we will be healthy and happy. If we are ignorant of the Natural Order we will be sickly and unhappy. Buddha said ignorance (to ignore), not sin, is the root cause of suffering. This is simple, clear, practical and realistic.

Most people simply do not realize that we are literally what we eat. If we eat large amounts of animal foods, refined foods, sugars of various kinds, preservatives, chemicals and colorings we will suffer from an endless list of illnesses. The idea that diet can cure illness is not accepted by the mainstream at all.

We must take responsibility for our health, and our very destiny. We must treat the CAUSE of our illnesses whether they be mental, emotional, physical or spiritual and not just try to remove the symptom. Today many of us go to the medical priests we call "doctors" and responsibility, instead of taking some of it on ourselves. We try to obliterate the symptom of our problem with surgery, drugs, radiation — and now microwaves and lasers — instead of looking at the cause of our suffering. It is only by dealing with the cause that we can be well again. You cannot be well just by treating the symptom and not knowing what caused this symptom to manifest. You cannot be well by giving the responsibility to any health professional whether traditional, allopathic, or naturopathic. You cannot get well by throwing money at your problems no matter how wealthy you are. You cannot get well by being butchered, poisoned and irradiated, microwaved and laseredYou can get well by aligning yourself with the Infinite Order and making better food choices, taking supplements that work, balancing your hormones, fasting regularly and by getting regular exercise. This is what natural health is all about.

Chapter 1: What is Macrobiotics?

The word "macrobiotic" comes from the Greek words "macro" or great and "bios" or life. Hippocrates (the Father of Medicine) and Herodotus used this method of eating natural foods to regain health and to treat their patients. This way of eating was popularized in Europe and America in the 1960's during the Psychedelic Era among the young people at the time. George Ohsawa was the main source of information with his books "Zen Macrobiotics" and "You Are All Sanpaku" William Dufty and his "Sugar Blues" also was popular. Then along came Michio Kushi, Herman Aihara and other writers. These few books had an immense influence — which is still very strong today — simply because this means of healing works. Their claims, that you could cure cancer and other terminal illnesses proved to be true.

One can certainly wonder how a man George Ohsawa showed up here in America with no money, no credentials or anything but his dream, and has had such a tremendous influence on American society over three decades later, and long after his death. There is an old saying, "one man plus truth equals an army". This is how George did it; he was merely a messenger for a very important message that people were ready to receive. His unsophisticated little paperback books became more and more popular as people found that they made sense and his advice really worked. The people who changed their way of life got the results he promised; the ones with illnesses were cured by changing their direction.

The underlying theory is really very simple. Its essence is simplicity. Thoreau said, "simplify, simplify, simplify." A macrobiotic diets consists of whole grains as its main, principal food. Most green and yellow vegetables are eaten. Beans are an important staple. Soups, salads, local fruit, and seafood are consumed in moderation. Tropical foods from hot climates such as bananas, citrus fruit, mangoes and the like are avoided. Nightshade family vegetables containing potatoes, tomatoes (tomatoes are botanically classed as fruits), peppers and eggplants are avoided as well as vegetables high in oxalic acid. Basically no sweeteners are used including honey and maple syrup. Just because a food is palatable this does not mean it is suited for us to eat. There are many foods that do not support a long and healthy life. On a macrobiotic diet, one drinks pure water or herb tea and eats only two meals a day. There is no meat, dairy, milk, poultry or eggs eaten. If one wants to be a vegetarian the seafood is left out. You always adapt to your genetics, the climate and the seasons. This in a few sentences is what comprises the macrobiotic way of eating which is always adaptable and flexible for each person.

In current Western religions, except a few like the Seven Day Adventists, dietetic principles are almost completely ignored. Even the Catholics have given up the practice of not eating meat on Fridays. In original Christianity and with within some modern Buddhists and Hindus factions such principles are integral. In Japan today this type of eating is called shojin ryori and is still popular in the countryside (but not the city) culture. Our biology and physiology are ignored instead of cared for. The teachings of the ancient religions always taught us that the body is a holy temple of the spirit and schooled us in the importance of healthful eating and drinking as well as avoiding harmful habits like coffee and alcohol. The Code of Manu, the Bible, the Canon of the Yellow Emperor, I Ching, Tao te Ching, Bhagavad Gita and Charak Samita all spoke of taking care of our earthly abode of consciousness, our physical body. You must be your own doctor; you must take responsibility for your health and happiness; you must heal yourself when ill. Be responsible for your own life.

Happy societies are based on millions of happy individuals. Imagine if the 6 billion people on this earth ate and drank and lived in harmony with the Divine Order. This planet would be all we have dreamed it could be. Our health and happiness are determined by our judgment, by our awareness and our faith in the Infinite. With good judgment we are happy and healthy. Macrobiotics is an art and there are no rules to follow. There are principles to lead us but no rules we must obey. Instead of structure there is flow. As the Zen master Lin Chi said, "At one stroke I forgot all my knowledge! There is no need for any discipline; for, move as I will, I always manifest the Tao." Macrobiotics is a deep understanding of the Ultimate Ground of Being that underlies all of existence. Above all, this is practical, pragmatic, logical, rational, sensible, based on common sense, and relates to the most everyday and mundane aspects of our lives, including washing the dishes and driving to work. The more we understand the Order of the Universe the more we harmonize with it and eat the foods that are best for us. As artists we create our own lives and design our own lifestyles by living in harmony with universal laws. We become our own doctors and follow the admonition, "physician, heal thyself." As we become more aware we gain freedom, health, happiness, creativity and spiritual realization. We take full and total responsibility for our lives and do not blame conditions, circumstances or people for our faults, limitations, problems and unhappiness. Look at your life....are you happy with it? Your life is exactly the way you made it and you are free to change it any way you choose in your heart. In your innermost being you do not really want to be a famous actor or actress, a powerful and influential politician, a billionaire business magnate, a legendary sports figure or other such meaningless fantasy?

Our overall attitude should be one of THANKFULNESS and being grateful for all we have been given, not taking anything for granted. We should always be thankful just for being incarnated in physical bodies and being alive on this earth. It is very rare to be given the gift of being alive in human form. Life is a brief flash of light in the cosmos and we have been given this chance to live anyway we want to and be anything we want to be. Always be thankful simply for being alive on this earth as a sentient, aware being.

The traditional way to talk about the whole grain based diet is the ten levels of eating with 100% whole grains at the top and 10% whole grains at the bottom. Let's try another way. The chart below gives percentages of each food group allowed for a specific regime.

#	grains/beans	vegs/soup	salad/fruit	animal
7	100%			
6	90%	10%		
5	80%	20%		
4	70%	30%		
3	60%	40%		
3	60%	30%	10% or	10%
2	50%	50%		
2	50%	40%	10% or	10%
2	50%	30%	20%	
2	50%	30%	10%	10%
1	40%	30%	20%	10%

Looking at this one could get the idea that we should eat diet #7 with 100% whole grains for ideal health when, in truth, we could only eat such a diet temporarily to heal and cleanse. Such a

11

regimen is seriously lacking in vitamins such as A and C and many B vitamins, minerals, and plant nutrients such as sterols, lignans, etc. Only 50-60% of our diet should be whole grains as our principal food. Diet #6 is also a temporary cleansing diet. Diet #5 is getting more practical but still far too limited except for temporary healing and cleansing. Diet #4 is a healthful, although very austere, diet that is more suited for people in monasteries or retreats. Dried beans are included with grains for simplicity and because they are so close as principal foods. Soup should consist of vegetables along with grains and beans in any combination. In Japanese macrobiotics the diet allowed only 5% to be soup but no reasons were given. A daily bowl of hot flavorful soup before dinner (and lunch as well) every day allows you to eat less food and feel full on less calories. Soups are no different from regular food as long as you CHEW the solids in your soup and do not swallow unchewed vegetables, grains and beans.

Diet #3 is a practical diet for the vegetarian with 60% grains, 30% vegetables and beans and 10% salads and fruits. Diet #2 is a practical diet for one who eats seafood. Actually diets #3 and #2 are the ideal way to eat every day and will, in fact, cure so called "incurable" illnesses such as cancer. Yes, you can cure disease while eating Diet #2 with 10% seafood. When we get to Diet #1 this is a less than ideal way to eat although certainly much superior to what the average person in America eats generally. Seafood should be limited to 10%. You can eat fresh salad regularly as long as you use a light and healthy dressing. You can eat up to 10% local fruit especially in the summer, but you really don't need fruit at all especially in winter. You'll see why this is true in Chapter 7 on Fruits and Sugars. Desserts are a temporary transition to healthy eating and are not part of your meal. Desserts are mostly an unnecessary Western custom and not part of a healthy lifestyle even if made with honey, fruit syrup, amazake or other natural sweetener.

Chapter 2: Yin and Yang

No book on macrobiotics would be complete without talking about yin and yang. Ohsawa called this "our guiding compass," as using this principle showed us right direction in our daily lives. In Oriental philosophy this is the unifying principle where the interplay of opposites is central. Yin is the feminine, cold, contracting violet energy while yang is the masculine, hot and expanding red energy. Together the universe and everything in it is made, preserved and dissolved. The universe we live in is not solid at all like we think, but rather an energy dance of vibrations. Existence is without beginning or end and beyond space and time and ever changing. Yin and yang are relative terms and not absolutes. Everything has both forces in it and nothing is purely yin or purely yang. The most yang substance has yin at its heart while the most yin substance has yang at its heart.

This is a very good way to look at the foods we eat in that a balance of yin and yang forces should prevail. Too much yin or too much yang ends up in sickness and ill health. You cannot balance yin and yang by going to extremes such as eating a very yin food like candy and then eating a very yang food like beef. You cannot cook tomatoes with salt for a long time to make them yang as the chemical constitution will remain the same basically. Balance means to eat proper foods in the right amounts so that a natural equilibrium prevails.

To get an idea of how this applies to what we eat the most yin to yang goes from yin drugs - sugars - alcohol - yeast - oil — fruit – yin dairy - nuts - water - sea vegetables - green and yellow vegetables – beans - grains – seafood – yang dairy - poultry - meat – eggs – salt - yang drugs. (Dairy products can be yang like hard cheese or yin like yogurt, and drugs can be yin like stimulants or yang like opiates). Please look at this chain of food from yin to yang very carefully and memorize it. It is obvious that vegetables, beans and grains are the basis of our diet. This gives you an idea of how to avoid the extremes in order to balance your body, mind, health and life. You cannot balance yourself by eating, for example, yogurt and fish and expecting them to cancel each other out. You can see in our present society where ill health comes from extreme intake of sweeteners of various type and animal products as the main staples. Colors go from yin ultraviolet

13

– violet – indigo – blue – green – yellow – brown – orange – red - yang infrared.

You can take this too far however and the originators certainly did. A perfect example is cherry tomatoes. These are small (yang), round (yang) and red (yang) but are one of the top ten allergenic foods on earth and chemically very yin. Whether you eat big, pear shaped yellow tomatoes or red cherry tomatoes makes very little difference in that most people simply are biologically incompatible with them and will react negatively to their regular intake. Too much concern about what is yin and what is yang and how to make yin foods more yang and yang foods more yin becomes more like arguing about how many angels can dance on the head of a pin than eating a balanced diet.

Yin and yang are always relative.

Whatever has a beginning has an end.

No two things are identical.

Oneness always manifests itself at all times as two forces we can call yin and yang.

Yin and yang are always changing into each other.

Yin attracts yang and yang attracts yin.

Yin repels yin and yang repels yang.

Nothing is only yin or only yang; everything is composed of both yin and yang together.

Nothing is balanced and static; everything is made up of dynamic and unequal portions of yin and yang.

The bigger the front, the bigger the back.

All antagonisms are, in reality, complementary.

The entire universe is unchanging, limitless, infinite, constant and omnipotent.

Your worst enemy is your best friend and will teach you more than anyone else.

Every experience in your life is exactly what you need at that moment and must be learned or it will be repeated.

Chapter 3: Whole Grains

Whole grains are literally the staff of life. Whole grains have been the staple of most civilizations since man mastered the art of agriculture over ten thousand years ago. The word "cereal" comes from the goddess Ceres. When man learned how to grow his own food, and not merely hunt and gather, he gained freedom for the first time. This was the major defining difference between cave people at the mercy of natural forces and people who forged their own destiny. Americans and Europeans today no longer eat many whole grains, however, and haven't for a long time. The rice is white, the bread is white, the cornmeal is de-germed, the cold cereal is refined, the flour is white and we have all but forgotten about oats, barley, buckwheat, millet and rye.

Why base your diet on whole grains? This has been the staple food for mankind for thousands of years and rightly so. Let's use extremes to make a point. If you ate nothing but red meat for a month what effects would it have? Ketosis, high cholesterol and triglycerides, bad body and mouth odor, a general feeling of malaise, physical weakness and other problems. If you ate only fruit for one month, how would you fare? Your blood glucose metabolism would become extremely disrupted, and a severe lack of nutrition and a dangerous sugar overload may occur. Eat just eggs and poultry? Results are very similar to meat but worse, since so many people have allergies to poultry and eggs. With just green and yellow vegetables, you would lose weight and lack protein and their nutrients, but would certainly feel great and look better; although you cannot continue on such a regimen. Eat just whole grains? You would feel and look wonderful, your mind would be clear, you would be full of energy and sharp, your body would be cleansed, your body fat would fall, many illnesses and conditions would be healed, but long term, you would lack vitamin A and certain other vitamins and minerals and other nutrients, that are found in beans and green and yellow vegetables. Clearly whole grains are our principal food.

The normal American diet involves eating twice the protein we need every day, five times the fat, as well as twice the calories. The idea of "protein deficiency" rarely exists and the actual reality is protein overload. The average whole grain contains about 8% high quality protein, which is readily bioavailable, of high quality with a wide variety of amino acids. When you eat beans regularly you will have an even wider variety of amino acids. The idea of lacking certain amino acids and having "incomplete" proteins is not based on science at all. You will get plenty of complete protein on a macrobiotic diet even if you choose to be a vegetarian and eat no seafood.

Let's start with **wheat**. Nearly all the wheat eaten in America is in the form of white flour. Even the whole wheat bread in the grocery stores is often filled with preservatives and is too puffed with air. Most bakeries do not sell real whole wheat bread, but rather "wheat bread" with white flour in it. You should be able to find a natural foods store or bakery that sells the real thing. Whole wheat breads vary quite a bit according to weight, water content, slice thickness and amount of oil added, but a typical slice has about 70 calories and 13% fat calories. You can find very good whole wheat breads or bake them yourself if you have the time. Most all the various pastas are made from white flour or a mixture of white and whole wheat flours, but you can readily find whole wheat pasta now in most chain grocery stores in a wide variety of types. Two ounces of dry whole wheat spaghetti is about 200 calories and when cooked contain only about 5% fat calories and will weigh about six ounces when drained al dente.

Bulgur wheat is whole wheat that has been soaked to expand it and then dried so it cooks more quickly. This retains most of the whole grain nutrition, contains only about 152 calories per cup cooked and a mere 3% fat calories, but it is not well known here. Couscous is nearly always a refined grain and not a good choice and should only be eaten occasionally in Mideastern restaurants. Look for whole wheat couscous in natural health stores for regular use. Whole wheat tortillas are best made at home with a simple ten dollar tortilla press since they are so difficult to find even in Latin grocery stores. Commercial cold cereals are rarely made with whole wheat and the few that are have sugar added to them. Fortunately it is easy to find good whole grain cold cereals even in chain groceries and not just natural food stores. A typical one has only about 120 calories per cup (30 g) dry. You'll rarely find whole wheat products when you go out to eat. Yes, there are occasional uses for unbleached white flour at times as a thickener in white sauces and soups, but not to replace whole wheat flour in breads and such.

It is true you should eat more steamed grains rather than flour products like bread and noodles. Traditional macrobiotics

16

recommends sour dough bread as if this is somehow not leavened with yeast. All risen bread is still based on yeast, wild or otherwise. The only unleavened "bread" is really a matzoh cracker. Yes, yeast is very yin, but it is completely dead after baking and you are getting very little cooked yeast proteins in a slice of bread. You should find heavy dense loaves that weigh about two pounds for a loaf that is about eight inches long and four inches high.

Whole unprocessed grains have a long shelf life while retaining their nutrition. Once ground into flour, however, they oxidize and lose their valuable nutrients. Ideally one should grind their own flour, but this is not practical for most people. It is best to buy refrigerated, fresh ground bread or pastry (without the gluten) flour in a natural food store if possible. If not, buy your flour in the grocery store and keep it refrigerated. The reason white flour does not need to be refrigerated is that the oils and nutrients have been so refined out of it and there is little else to lose. Definitely you want to eat more steamed grains than flour products such as noodles and bread as a general rule.

Brown rice is sold in most any grocery and Oriental grocery store now. Some Chinese restaurants offer brown rice with your meal if you request it. It is worthwhile buying 25 pound bags of organically grown brown rice since many chemicals are used to raise regular rice. You can buy exotic brown rice like jasmine and basmati if you're willing to pay up for them. A big deal was made of eating the short grain variety rather than the long grain variety, since the short grain is supposedly more yang. Most people who eat natural foods seem to prefer the short grain variety, but it really doesn't make much difference if you buy a good organically grown rice. You can also find short grain "sweet rice" but it is laborious to cook correctly and takes a long time. The taste is very different and the best use for it is in desserts. Brown rice pasta is popular now, but you have to cook it carefully (never too long) and cool it off once it is cooked. Brown rice flour is available and is mostly used for baking. You can find brown rice cold cereals as well as cold cereals that use brown rice in the mix of whole grains. Rice is most versatile and can be used in many ways in very different types of dishes. A lot of people choose to eat brown rice as their staple food as they feel it simply tastes better than the other grains. One cup of cooked brown rice has about 173 calories and 5% fat calories. Urban people in Japan, Thailand, Viet Nam, China, Korea and other Asian countries eat white rice as a tradition and it can be very difficult to find brown rice in city restaurants.

Wild rice, like buckwheat is not botanically a grain. Wild rice is really a grass with a strong flavor and is pricey compared with brown rice. This is a perfectly good food, but you may want to use it to flavor your brown rice and other grains rather than eat it by itself as the taste is simply too assertive and strong. This makes a good addition to your other grains and adds variety and flavor. It has even less calories than brown rice as it contains only 3% fat calories.

Corn as a vegetable, is still eaten whole on the cob. Frozen corn is acceptable out of season. Whole cornmeal white or yellow is popular, but make sure it is *whole* corn and not "degermed" with the nutrition removed. A fancy word for corn meal mush is "polenta" which is served in some of the finest restaurants especially Northern Italian ones. If you have never had polenta, it is very easy and quick to fix and quite good as well as inexpensive. Just take 1 cup of corn meal and three cups of water or vegetable stock and cook for about ten minutes. You can use one cup of non-dairy milk and two cups of water to make it creamy. Corn grits are a Southern staple but have been degermed and are not a whole grain. I have never been able to find whole corn grits and cannot verify they really exist. Anything labeled "hominy" is degermed unfortunately. Good corn chips that are baked rather than fried are an excellent whole grain food. Latins use harina masa or finely ground corn flour rather than coarse meal, but be sure this is ground from whole corn and not degermed. An ear of corn has about 89 calories and 10% fat calories and is equal to a half cup of fresh or frozen corn kernels. A quarter cup of corn meal (30 grams) has 100 calories and 10% fat calories and cooked with three quarters of a cup of water or stock would make a large serving of polenta.

Oats are rarely eaten now except as oatmeal for breakfast. Too often oatmeal is instant or quick cooking. Be sure to buy the "old fashioned" oatmeal as it cooks in a few minutes. Oat groats and steel cut oats are other choices. Very few people use oat flour, but it goes well in breads and baking. Oat flakes also go very well in baking. Some whole grain cold cereals include oats in them. This is a very yang cereal with a high oil content that grows in cold regions and very good for cold climates and during winter months. A cup of cooked oatmeal has 145 calories and 12% fat calories so it is especially good for cold weather. It's a shame such a fine flavorful grain is generally limited only to breakfast cereal.

Buckwheat is not botanically a grain but certainly is rightly considered a grain for practical purposes. You can buy buckwheat groats in the grocery store. Very few people eat buckwheat groats anymore, but they are quite good and mix well with other grains. Try half buckwheat and half brown rice for a change. Buckwheat cooks very quickly. You can find hot cereals made of buckwheat as well. An emphasis was made in macrobiotics about eating buckwheat noodles or "soba". Go to an Oriental store and you will find all the buckwheat noodles to be filled with white flour. Buckwheat lacks gluten to hold it together and must be mixed with wheat flour. I have never found buckwheat noodles made with whole wheat flour for some reason. They are very expensive and simply have no advantage over whole wheat or brown rice pastas. Buckwheat groats are delicious, can be mixed with other grains and very nutritious especially in winter as they are very yang and grown in cold climates such as Canada.

Rye is not commonly eaten today except mixed with white flour in rye bread. Rye pasta is available though. Nearly all rye is used to make whiskey. Rye has a strong and distinctive flavor with no gluten and cannot stand alone in bread. There are a few hot cereals made with rye, but they are not very widely sold. When you make your own whole grain bread be sure to make some rye bread with one third rye and two thirds whole wheat flour along with caraway seeds and cornmeal.

Millet is a popular staple in some African countries but not very popular here. You can buy whole millet and try it and discover a whole new grain as it is very available and inexpensive. It is very easy to steam millet and it can be mixed with your rice for variety. You can add millet flour to homemade bread as well. You'll often find this in multi-grain breads. A cup of cooked millet reportedly contains about 287 calories and 6% fat calories which seems high because cooked millet does not contain much water and is very filling. This is a staple food in some countries yet not popular here in America, but is a fine grain to eat with a lot of nutrition.

What about **spelt, teff** and **quinoa** (KEEN-wa)? These are ancient grains, can be hard to find and rather expensive compared to other grains. Try these for variety as they do differ in taste. You

19

will find bread, baked goods and pastas containing these. As they become more common the price will come down.

If you could eat only one food to stay alive your best choice would be a whole grain as you could thrive on this for a long time. Whole grains are the ideal food and should be the basis of your diet, your principal food. Whole grains are easily digested and leave no toxins in the body during their metabolism. They contain all the protein you need, are very low in fat, high in fiber, low in calories and very concentrated in nutrition. Whole grains are also the best food to regulate your blood sugar. Blood sugar dysmetabolism — both low and high — is epidemic in Western societies. This is largely because we have forgotten whole grains as our main source of nutrition, which is the central food of the macrobiotic way of eating.

Some grains can be successfully sprouted including barley, buckwheat, rice, wheat, millet, oats and triticale. You can find these in natural food stores or easily sprout them at home. Try these for variety and taste.

Get some cookbooks on how to cook grains in a variety of international styles and you'll find they quickly become an immensely enjoyable principal food you look forward to every day. It can be difficult at first to use whole grains as your principal food when you haven't been used to them. Once you learn to cook them in flavorful ways they will become the center of your every meal. You'll come to love whole grains as the center of every meal and look forward to enjoying them in a variety of ways.

Chapter 4: Beans

Beans are a wonderful food that feeds much of the world. Dried beans should be a staple in your diet. You will come to enjoy them very much as you learn to cook and flavor them in international styles. In affluent societies such as ours they are often looked at as food for poor people. Go to the store and buy some pintos, lentils, black-eyed peas, chili beans, black beans, northern, pink, chickpeas, kidney, limas, navy and cannellini beans. Now go to a Latin market and you'll find beans you've probably never heard of. Buy one of each variety like pigeon peas and favas and go home and try them. Go to a gourmet store or search the internet and you'll really find some interesting ones like appaloosa, calypso, Christmas limas, cranberry, European soldiers, yellow eyed peas, white emergo, trout, tongues of fire, Swedish brown beans, snowcaps, scarlet runners, Spanish Tolosanas, French flageolets, French navy, Jackson wonders, piebald, provence, rattlesnake and rice beans.

Go to the library and get some international cookbooks and see how the cooks of the world prepare their beans. Bean soups, refried beans, pasta and beans, bean dips, bean salads, and bean spreads like hummus show their versatility. Some beans can be sprouted especially soy, mung, lentil, green and yellow peas, chickpeas and adzuki beans. Try adding bean thread to your soups and stir fry's. Well-cooked beans are anything but food for Third World and poor people. The early macrobiotic teachers emphasized adzuki beans only because the Japanese actually eat very few types of beans in their diet. Enjoy all varieties of beans cooked in various international styles with good herbal flavorings.

Beans are very high in protein, vitamins, minerals and plant nutrients like lignans and sterols, but without the calories or the fat. People who start eating beans sometimes have excess gas, but this basically goes away as the body gets acclimated to eating them and your intestines become healthier. There are digestive enzymes such as Beano® (alpha-galactosidase) available if you want to take them but it isn't necessary. To give you an idea of the nutritional profile of common beans here are some basic facts (per half cup cooked):

Bean	Calories	% Fat Calories	% Protein
Chick Peas	120	4	20
Kidney	112	1	20
Lentils	115	1	26
Pinto/Calico	117	1	19
Lima	111	1	20
Blackeyed	100	2	17
Yellow Soybeans	139	1	29
Red beans	100	1	20
Black beans	113	4	23
Navy beans	129	1	21
Northern beans	104	1	19
Pink beans	125	1	20
Cannelli	125	1	20
Fava	100	2	30
Split peas	15	1	24

It can take 2 to 3 hours to cook beans so you can cook up a pound bag and freeze half of them if you want to. Remember to bring them to a boil, turn off the heat and let them hotsoak for a few hours before cooking. Do not add salt until after they have soaked. Never add baking soda to make them cook quicker as some cookbooks suggest. Adding vegetables such as garlic, carrots, onions, leeks and celery makes them more colorful and interesting. Be sure to use your favorite herbs, spices and flavorings to make them even more delicious.

What about tofu, which is so popular? This is a very versatile food, but a very refined one missing most of the nutrition and is over 50% fat calories. It cannot be sautéed as it absorbs oil like a sponge. It certainly does have uses but this is just not a staple food. Tempeh as a whole food is a much better choice as it is a whole food with all the nutrition of the soybean.

When you learn to use and cook beans in new and creative ways you'll come to enjoy them as a regular part of your diet. Beans are next to grains as a principal food due to their high nutrition, good protein, high fiber, low fat content and low calories.

Chapter 5: Vegetables

It seems most Americans are rather bored by green and yellow vegetables. This is really due to the poor cooking methods used to prepare them. Most restaurants, except home-style eateries in the south, barely serve them and fast food restaurants serve almost none. Even gourmet restaurants often only offer one single vegetable du jour. The way green and yellow vegetables are cooked and served is a very good reason more people aren't attracted to them. Many people still buy vegetables including leafy ones in cans. Some frozen vegetables are very tasty and full of nutrition and can be acceptable in winter when they are out of season. Fortunately, we have a wide variety of fresh vegetables available all year round here in America. Most people eat their vegetables boiled until they're soggy and then flavored with butter, salt and pepper. The Asians are the premier vegetable cooks and the usual preparation is a stir fry with lots of good flavors added such as ginger, garlic, soy sauce, sherry, oyster sauce, dark sesame oil, black bean sauce, chili sauce and others. Get some Chinese, Vietnamese and Thai cookbooks for interesting ways to flavor your favorite vegetables.

One could easily get the idea from reading the early macrobiotic books that Diet #7 as stated previously, is ideal and the more grains and less vegetables you eat the better. This is a big misunderstanding and eating only whole grains is a very temporary regimen for people with serious illness. It is important to eat lots of fresh green and yellow vegetables with your grains and beans. You can eat as much as fifty percent of fresh vegetables with a minimum of twenty five per cent. You'll eat more vegetables in the summer when you need lighter food, and fewer calories and less in the winter when you need heavier food and more calories.

Let's take a look at some of the many good vegetables we can eat. Asparagus, artichoke, bok choy, bush and pole beans, bean sprouts, beets, broccoli, Brussels sprouts, red and green cabbage, Chinese cabbage, carrots, cauliflower, celery, Swiss chard (occasionally), cucumbers, garlic, edible gourds, endive, collard and mustard greens, kale, kohlrabi, leeks, lettuce (many varieties other than iceberg), lotus root, many types of mush rooms, okra, onions, parsnips, peas, snow peas, various pumpkins, radish, daikon radish, rutabaga, salsify, Malabar spinach and New Zealand spinach (Tetragonia not Spinacia), green and yellow squashes, various winter squashes, green beans, sweet potatoes (which are not yams), turnips and watercress.

The older macrobiotic books also kept recommending such hard to obtain and expensive vegetables like adzuki beans, burdock root, Hokkaido pumpkin, mountain potatoes (jijeno) and other such Japanese foods that just aren't normally available in America and are expensive. These have no advantage over the vegetables that are readiily available and can be very hard to find even in Asian food stores.

A word about **onions and garlic;** onions and garlic must always be cooked to evaporate the irritating volatile oils and must never be eaten raw. Raw garlic and onions are used as natural insecticides due to their irritating nature. Certain yogic systems do not allow onions and garlic as they are considered too "rajastic" — stimulating and disturbing to the body. Some people will be allergic and biologically incompatible with these vegetables and should not eat them. If they cause indigestion please drop both of them from your diet. It has been verified in clinical studies that for most people, the substances in garlic have been shown to have healing properties, although some people may be allergic.

Raw Vegetables: You rarely see raw vegetables recommended in traditional macrobiotics. It is true that people on an all-raw food diet quickly become very sickly and need to stop such a regimen, but raw foods are part of eating well especially in the summer when lighter fare is needed. Most vegetables are simply inedible when eaten raw and need light cooking to make them palatable. The idea of "pressing" and salting your salad greens before eating them is very unnecessary and ruins crisp lettuce and other raw vegetables. A small salad makes a wonderful and colorful addition to a meal especially in summer when lighter fare is eaten. The real concern is finding a low-fat or no-fat dressing to go on it. Many Latins have a custom of simply squeezing lime juice over their salad and do not use creamy dressings at all. Asians flavor their salad greens with such things as vinegar and sesame seeds.

Salted and salt pickled vegetables: These are popular in cold remote areas. Inhabitants living in monasteries in cold climates use this method in winter since they have no access to fresh vegetables. The salt overload from such foods is just not necessary. Pickled vegetables are still popular in Asian areas where there is no refrigeration. There is just no reason to eat pick-led vegetables including the popular preserved daikon radish. It is far preferable to eat fresh vegetables especially since a wide variety of them are available all year round. There are times when frozen vegetables are fine in winter; there is a loss of texture in these, but no loss of nutrition.

Sea vegetables: Commonly referred to as "seaweeds"c traditional macrobiotics recommends we eat these very nutritious vegetables from the ocean. Seaweeds such as nori, kombu and hiziki, are the best source of minerals we can eat and can be found at oriental grocery stores. Unfortunately Americans have never cultivated much of a taste for them. Most people refuse to eat seaweeds except maybe when they eat nori wrapped sushi. Buy some of the various sea vegetables and at least try them in small amounts. You only need a tablespoonful at meals and it makes an elegant garnish.

To change your view of vegetables so you can see how delicious they are, go get some international cookbooks and see how the chefs of the world prepare different vegetables. Modify any recipes if possible that sound good, but don't use the ingredients you want. Most recipes can be adapted to be healthful.

Methods of cooking include tempura used extensively in Japanese restaurants. Unfortunately because of the cooking method used, these vegetables contain very high in oil content no matter how skillfully cooked. This certainly adds to the flavor, but is not a heathful way to eat vegetables regularly. Tempura should be reserved for special occasions. You can also use a pressure cooker to accelerate cooking time, but very few people do. The idea that this makes food more yang is technically true, but rather unimportant.

Notice that sprouts weren't included in traditional Japanese macrobiotics. There are many seeds that can be sprouted to add taste and variety to your vegetables, salads and sandwiches. Many kinds of sprouts are available in grocery stores now and making sprouts at home is easy and fun. Just some of the vegetable seeds that can be successfully sprouted are alfalfa, cabbage, broccoli, Brussels sprouts, cauliflower, kale, chia, cress, radish, and fenugreek.

If you want to lose weight and eat less calories simply eat more healthy green and yellow vegetables temporarily. Your diet should contain fifty per cent whole grains as your principal food, but to lose weight you can temporarily eat less grain, less beans and more green and yellow vegetables, but no seafood and add local fruit at a ratio of no more than ten percent. Vegetable soup is an excellent alternative to strict fasting for up to a week to lose an impressive amount of weight while never being hungry. Just make soups from your favorite vegetables with no grains or beans and flavor these fully. Vegetables have less calories than any other food group. Vegetable soup can become a partial fast with a healthful side benefit from the very low calorie intake.

Calorie Content of Common Vegetables
(100 grams)

Artichoke	26
Asparagus	26
Beets	31
Broccoli	18
Brussels sprouts	32
Cabbage	27
Carrots	52
Cauliflower	27
Celery	14
Cucumber	9
Kale	33
Leeks	52
Lettuce	35
Mushrooms	40
Onions	24
Radishes	17
Squash, Summer	14
Squash, Winter	25
Turnip Greens	24

Chapter 6:
Seafood, Meat, Poultry and Dairy

For health or ethical reasons, you can be a vegetarian if you choose to. The macrobiotic diet can include seafood of most any type in moderation, especially in winter and in cold climates. Moderation would mean four to six ounce portions several times a week. Or you can choose to eat only plant-based foods. It is best to eat lower calorie, lower fat, white, fleshed fish like cod, perch, flounder, grouper, sole, halibut, haddock and other varieties. Shellfish such as crab, shrimp, scallops, clams, oysters and lobster are also good choices. Minimize or avoid the high fat white fish like catfish, orange roughy and turbot. The same applies to red fleshed fish like tuna, mackerel, salmon and swordfish. It is a biological and physiological fact that our teeth and digestive systems are designed to eat small amounts of animal food, and seafood is the healthiest animal food to eat. Fat content varies dramatically from 7% to 52%. You can eat a 3 1/3 ounce (100 g) portion of seafood and generally get less than 100 calories, plus it is very filling on a caloric basis.

There is no reason to eat red meat such as beef, pork and lamb or wild meats such as venison, rabbit and squirrel for many reasons. Americans eat twice the protein they need which causes very negative conditions in the body, such as high blood urea and other negative parameters of our bloodstream. Excess protein creates a toxic environment in our intestines. Animal proteins are very different from vegetable proteins and like animal fats, are highly correlated with many diseases such as diabetes, arthritis and cancers of various types. Proteins are not a good energy source as they have to be broken down in steps and leave toxic byproducts in our blood. Complex carbohydrates are a direct energy source on the other hand and do not leave unwanted byproducts as they are digested. We only need about 0.6 grams of protein per kilogram of body weight so even a 154 pounds person only needs about 42 grams of protein daily. You get all the complete protein you need by eating a variety of whole grains, beans and vegetables and we do not need animal foods as a source of protein at all.

Poultry and eggs are two of the top ten allergenic foods known and these should be avoided. Trying not to eat poultry and eggs in western society can be very difficult, because they are almost everywhere, inexpensive and served in a variety of tasty ways. Some people eat eggs yet call themselves "vegetarians". It makes no difference whether an egg is organically produced or not or whether it is fertile or not as they are still eggs and as a macrobiotic, should not be eaten. Eggs are eggs. Whole eggs are 64% fat calories and contain a whopping 250 mg of cholesterol. Some people eat egg whites, but these are just as allergenic as the yolks and still made up of animal proteins. Poultry even steamed or broiled without the skin, is neither a healthy food nor even a low fat food.

Milk is the number one worst food allergen of all known foods. No other food is a universal allergen like milk and the products derived from milk. Whole milk is an amazing 48% fat calories. To learn more about the many reasons not to drink milk or eat dairy products visit the websites: www.milksucks.com or www.notmilk.com. Cow's milk is meant for calves — not human babies much less human adults.

Dairy products are eaten by some people who call themselves "vegetarians". Whether the milk and dairy products are organically produced or not, is beside the point and does not change the basic nature of them. Since dairy is not made from vegetables this is certainly not an accurate description. What is wrong with dairy products? They contain lactose and all adults of all races are lactose intolerant. Any biologist knows that all mammals lose the ability to produce the enzyme lactase soon after birth and weaning. Lactose (milk sugar) does not just pass through your digestive system like fiber, but also causes allergic reactions. There are a lot of other reasons not to eat dairy products even if you go to the trouble and expense of buying organic and low fat products. Alternatives to dairy include soy, oat, rice, and almonds so there is no reason to eat it. You can buy soy sour cream, soy yogurt, many flavors of meltable soy cheese and can make your own soy cream cheese by draining soy yogurt.

Yogurt is considered a "health food" by many people, but is anything but healthy. Yogurt contains twice the lactose of regular milk because milk powder is added to thicken it. Soy yogurts are available but do not taste as good, can be hard to find, are expensive and usually full of sugar. Hard cheeses contain little lactose (it is drawn off in the whey during processing), but are so full of saturated fat (over 70% in most varieties) and calories to make them poor food choices. Soy cheese is meltable, tastes like dairy cheese but is high in fat and should not be used regularly. Sour cream, cream, cream cheese and all the rest are very unhealthy foods to eat. Probably the least objectionable is low fat cottage cheese, as it has a minimum of lactose and fat, but has a lot of animal protein so there is really no excuse to eat it. Many people have been buying the low fat and no fat dairy products thinking these were "good for them".

Seafood is the best animal food to eat if you choose not to be a vegetarian. Seafood is best for men rather than women, for hard working people or those who exercise a lot and are physically active, in colder climates and in the colder seasons, as it is very yang. Seafood should be limited in hotter climates and in summertime. A small percent of people have a generalized allergy to fish and/or shellfish and this should be obvious if it exists, although there are hidden allergies. It is best to choose shellfish and light fleshed, low fat fish such as cod, flounder, sole and others over dark fleshed, high fat fish such as tuna, swordfish and salmon.

Regarding red meat there are two reasons not to eat cows, pigs, sheep, deer, chickens, turkeys and other animals. In Buddhism "ahimsa", or doing no harm, is a basic tenet. We do not need to kill any animals to be healthy and we do this only for sensory pleasure. If you are going to eat meat or poultry, be honest with yourself about the life you are taking. If you had to personally kill and butcher a cow, a pig, some chickens and turkeys and especially a veal calf or a young lamb would you still be eating them? If you were directly responsible for their death how much meat and poultry would you be eating? The second reason is biological. In macrobiotics fish and shellfish are eaten in moderation if one chooses to do so. We are biologically equipped to include in our diets about one tenth animal foods. We have long digestive systems designed to basically eat grains, beans, vegetables and fruit and teeth to match this system.

There is no doubt that eating meat and poultry results in far more disease of every kind, less quality of life and a shorter lifespan. The longest-lived people on earth are the Okinawans who eat fish they and a very small amount of animal foods such as chicken and eggs. Their basic diet is excellent and they work hard physically even in old age.

Calories and Fat Calories in Common Seafood
(raw, 100 g)

Fish	Cal	Fat Cal.	Fish	Cal	Fat Cal.
Catfish	110	33	Halibut	103	19
Turbot	90	28	Flounder	84	7
Perch	89	11	Snapper	94	11
Cod	79	7	King crab	78	13
Swordrish	114	26	Blue Crab	82	11
Salmon	135	31	Clams	70	11
Mackerel	131	38	Mussels	81	23
Scallops	83	7	Mahi	80	7
Sea trout	97	31	Grouper	86	10
Lobster	106	10	Oysters	76	25
Sole	64	8	Ocean Perch	94	11
Tuna	135	30	Squid	86	12
Rockfish	89	11	Shrimp	100	10
Kingfish	100	26	Carp	119	40
Haddock	100	7	Herring	149	52
Monkfish	71	14	Pollack	86	10
Sea Bass	90	19	Roughy	119	49
Shark	123	31	Croaker	99	27

A study was done at the Oregon Health Sciences University and published in Circulation in 1993 (vol. 88, p. 2771-9) on milk intake and the death from coronary heart disease — the largest killer of all of both men and women. The populations of 40 different countries were studied. You can see the yearly death rate approaches zero per hundred thousand in people who drink no or almost no milk. The people who drink the most milk had the highest death rate. Finland had literally one thousand people die from heart disease every single year, who drank only one cup of milk per 1,000 calories of food intake. This chart is based on millions of people in forty different countries and simply cannot be disputed.

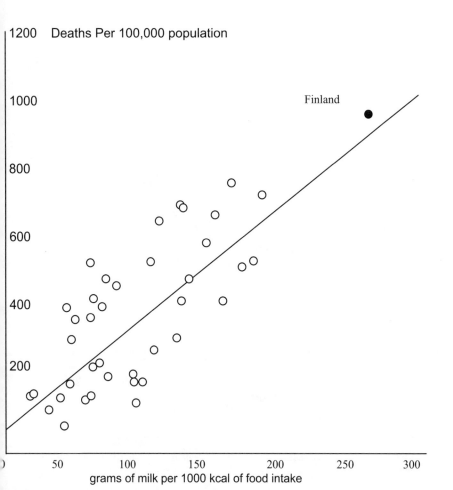

1200   Deaths Per 100,000 population

1000   Finland

800

600

400

200

50   100   150   200   250   300
grams of milk per 1000 kcal of food intake

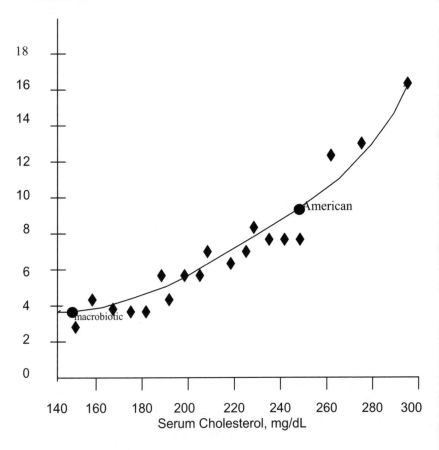

Age-adjusted Six-Year
Death Rate Per 1000

Serum Cholesterol, mg/dL

The MRFIT Study was one of the largest and longest of all human studies on heart and artery health. This chart is based on 361,662 people 35 to 57 years old studied for a period of 6 years.

You can see by the two round dots that people who eat macrobiotically and have an average total cholesterol level of about 150, have the fewest deaths of all from heart and artery disease. The average American has a cholesterol level of 250 and suffers about 250% more deaths every year. The lower your cholesterol the better and the only source of cholesterol is animal products like meat, poultry, eggs and dairy products. Seafood in moderation does not raise your cholesterol level.

Chapter 7: Fruits and Sugars

People are usually very surprised to find that in macrobiotics eating fruit is not recommended except in small amounts and only locally grown fruits. If you study a nutrition profile of most any fruit you will find it is basically just water, sugar and one or two vitamins with a little fiber. Fruit is a particularly poor source of nutrients and contains far too much sugar. If you will look at the two charts on the following pages you can see the scientific validation. Fruits generally have very little vitamins and almost no minerals in addition to being full of simple sugars. Please look at the two nutrition charts for common fruits like fructose and sucrose. Since you need 1,000 mg of calcium, 400 mg of magnesium, 18 mg of iron, 5 mg of copper, 2 mg of manganese, 15 mg of zinc, 120 mcg of chromium and 70 mcg of selenium daily you are getting biologically insignificant amounts of any minerals no matter how much fruit, or which fruit you eat.

The situation is hardly any better with vitamins. You are receiving no realistic amounts at all of vitamins E, K, thiamine, riboflavin, niacin, B-6, folic acid, B-12, pantothenic acid and biotin. In a few fruits you will get some vitamins A or C, and that's all.

Definitely fruit juice, fruit concentrate and dried fruits should be avoided, as these are concentrated sugars. Remember that all sugar is sugar and all sugar is "natural". Whether you use white sugar, brown sugar, raw sugar, molasses, honey, maple syrup, date sugar, fructose, corn syrup, cane sugar, maltose, or amazake you are still eating simple sugars and these are all basically the same. You need no fruit in your diet at all actually, and the only reason to eat it is for variety and taste as this is the least nutrient dense group of foods.

If you choose to include fruit in your diet pick temperate ones like plums, berries, peaches, cherries, apples, grapes and such. Do not eat tropical fruits like coconuts, guavas, mangos, papayas, bananas, avocados and others. This is discussed in the chapter on "Tropical and Nightshade Foods". The best time of year to include one serving of fruit a day in your diet is summer time when it is naturally available. Fruits are very yin and more appropriate in the yang summer time. The least appropriate time is in the winter when they are not naturally available at all. If you live in hot, yang sunny area like Southern Florida or Southern

33

California please do not rationalize this as a reason to eat a lot of fruit especially tropical fruit.

Most vegetarians, especially vegans, are addicted to simple sugars and eat far too much honey, dried fruits, fruit juices, raw sugar, maple syrup, tropical fruits, desserts, sodas and other sweets. They rationalize this by saying these are "natural sugars". There is no reason at all to eat desserts at the end of a meal. You'll be better off if you take the concept of "dessert" out of your dietary regimen. At first you may want some sweets, so get a natural dessert cookbook and learn how to make desserts out of whole grains and unsweetened fruit. Remember this is a temporary stage and not something to continue. Have you noticed that cultures like the Chinese, Thai, Koreans and Japanese do not understand the idea of having desserts at the end of the meal? This is a very good concept to adopt in your own life.

Diabetes (hyperglycemia), insulin resistance and other blood sugar disorders like hypoglycemia are epidemic in America. One big reason is the inordinate intake of about 125 pounds of various sugars per year in our diets. Imagine scarfing down more than two pounds of different sugars every week. Refined carbohydrates and excessive fat intake are two other reasons for this. Eating whole grains slowly releases glucose into our blood as it is needed. Doctors are still recommending harmful high protein diets for such people which, of course, ends up with them being on insulin and other prescription drugs to cover up the symptom. To eat a high protein diet you have to also eat a lot of saturated fat and cholesterol.

Adult onset diabetes is now widespread along with insulin resistance. Insulin resistance means the body produces enough insulin, but the cells don't metabolize it well. Get a glucose tolerance test (GTT) if you feel this may be affecting you, as the blood glucose may be normal. People who have low blood sugar or hypoglycemia, may experience symptoms such as constant hunger even after eating, weakness and fatigue, perspiring too much, yawning inappropriately and emotional swings.

VITAMIN CONTENT OF COMMON FRUITS

FRUIT	gr	A	C	E	K	Thia.	Rib.	Nia	B6	Fol.	B12	Pant.	Bio.
Apple	150	52	6	.90	0	.02	.01	.08	.05	3	0	.06	.90
Apricot	40	2612	10	.75	0	.03	.04	.60	.05	9	0	.24	0
Banana	150	81	9	.40	2	.05	.10	.50	.58	19	9	.26	4.40
Blueberry	140	100	13	0	0	.05	.05	.40	.04	64	0	.09	0
Cantaloupe	400	3220	42	.20	0	.04	.02	.60	.12	17	0	1.13	3.0
Grapes	150	100	4	0	0	.09	.06	.30	.11	4	0	.02	1.60
Oranges	180	200	53	.36	1	.09	.04	.30	.06	30	0	.25	1.90
Peaches	100	535	7	.90	8	.02	.04	1.0	.02	3	0	.17	1.70
Pears	75	20	4	.80	0	.02	.04	.10	.20	7	0	.07	.10
Pineapple	140	25	15	.15	0	.09	.04	.40	.08	11	0	.16	0
Plums	100	320	10	.70	0	.04	.10	.50	.18	2	0	.18	.10
Strawberry	150	27	57	.18	13	.02	.07	.20	.54	18	0	.34	4.0

MINERAL CONTENT OF COMMON FRUITS

FRUIT	grams	CaP	Mg	K	Na	Fe	Cu	Mn	Zn	Se	(mcg) Cr	(mcg)
Apple	150	7	7	5	115	1	.2	.04	.05	.04	.30	2
Apricots	40	14	19	12	296	1	.5	.04	.08	.26	0	0
Bananas	150	6	20	29	400	1	.3	.10	.15	.16	1	9
Blueberry	140	6	10	5	90	6	.2	.06	.30	.11	0	5
Cantaloupe	400	11	17	11	310	9	.2	.04	.04	.16	0	2
Grapes	150	1410	5	190	2	.3	.04	.72	.04	0	3	
Oranges	180	40	14	10	180	1	.1	.05	.03	.07	1.3	3
Peaches	100	5	12	7	200	1	.1	.07	.05	.14	.40	2
Pears	75	11	11	6	130	2	.3	.11	.08	.12	.60	2
Pineapple	140	7	7	14	110	1	.4	.11	1.7	.08	.60	0
Plums	100	4	10	7	172	2	.1	.04	.05	.10	0	2
Strawberry	150	14	19	10	170	1	.4	.12	.30	.13	0	3

Chapter 8: Other Diets

There are so many different diets that are popular now. With all this contradictory information how does one decide what really works and what doesn't? In one word —RESULTS. When you see people advocate a certain diet are they healthy and happy? Do they look good and feel good? Are they youthful in nature with lots of energy and a good disposition? "By their fruits shall ye know them" as the Bible tells us. Look at the RESULTS of all these other ways of eating. And look at the authors of the many different books. Most of these diet gurus are overweight, have high cholesterol, look older than their years — despite plastic surgery — and have a wide variety of illnesses they don't disclose. The whole grain based way of eating we call "macrobiotics" is the only way that has been proven here in the U.S. for over three decades with results of maximum health, staying slim and curing "incurable" illnesses. No other way of eating can say that.

The most popular diet in history is the so-called ketogenic diet, Paleolithic diet or "Atkins Diet" as proposed by Robert Atkins who fell over of cardiomyopathy in April of 2002 from following his own advice. He is the most popular diet author in history by far. This is proof that to be successful you merely need to tell people what they want to hear. Atkins tells people to eat all the meat, poultry, eggs, milk, butter, cheese, dairy products, vegetable oils and seafood they want to, but God help you if you eat any whole grains! To his credit he does advocate abstaining from simple sugars of any kind, refined grains like white flour or hydrogenated oils. This goes along with the "glycemic index" where all carbohydrates are considered equal. The buzzword "carbs" is used constantly to refer to any and all carbohydrates. Brown rice is the "same" as white sugar, oatmeal is the "same" as a Twinkie, and whole grain bread is "no different" than candy bars. Many otherwise intelligent people have fallen for this transparent pseudoscience. Anyone who can't tell the difference between whole grains and sugary junk food is obviously beyond help anyway and won't last long on a regimen like this.

It seems people never notice that the word "ketogenic" comes from the word "ketosis", a disease state! That's right — this diet is named after a condition of *sickness* where ketone bodies in the blood are excessive causing illness. "Ketogenic" means having a disease condition. Look up the word "ketosis" in your dictionary to see for yourself. The most popular diet in history is modeled after a disease state! This shows you that truth is always stranger than fiction doesn't it?

Another popular diet is the raw food diet, where everything you eat must be raw and uncooked. Cooking is "bad" because it destroys the enzymes in "live food." Food must be alive! You cannot cook anything, so if it doesn't taste good raw you just don't eat it. Obviously this limits most of your normal food choices. Some grains and beans can be sprouted however. This is an understandable reaction to a lifetime of eating meat, dairy products and overcooked foods. People who eat this way quickly become thin, weak, and sickly with bad skin and low immunity. The idea that cooking "kills" all your foods is silly. Cooking grains and beans is necessary to even eat them. Lightly cooking most of your green and yellow vegetables makes them taste better and makes them more digestible, not less digestible. Certainly you should eat some raw foods and some salads with your meals especially in warm climates and in summer. A strict diet of raw, uncooked foods will quickly convince you this is an irrational extreme that leads to debilitation. It is important to realize that cooking food makes it more digestible and this is what distinguishes us from animals, who are unable to cook their food. People who are ill often have difficulty in digesting raw foods and do much better when their food is minimally cooked.

Another diet that has been popular for years is the one based on your blood type. Unfortunately, your blood type has almost no relevance except when you need a blood transfusion. Since people are always looking for a simplistic answer, this has become amazingly popular. There are four basic blood types and you are supposed to base your diet on which one you are. Type O means you are a Meat Eater and should eat red meat, poultry, eggs and seafood as the basis of your diet and no whole grains or beans. Type A means you are a Vegetarian, but for some unknown reason the author just doesn't like wheat. This is the most intelligent of the diets obviously. Type B is the Nomad and you can eat pretty much anything you want to as the caveman did, especially dairy products. Type AB is the Enigma (only 5% of the population) and this combines the rules for both type A and B and you can eat a lot of eggs but no corn for some unknown reason. That this kind of foolishness has become so popular is an important insight to our current culture.

Food combining or the "fit for life" diet is based on the teachings of Herbert Shelton decades ago. Poor Herbert died prematurely of a horrible disease from following his own advice. With this diet you eat a lot of raw fruits, nuts and vegetables with a lot of scientifically unbased rules on not combining starches with proteins and other prohibitions. Harvey Diamond is currently reviving this and Tony Robbins adopted it for years before admitting how wrong he had been and how poorly he and his wife had fared on such a regimen.

The "zone" diet (controlling your zone of insulin values) or 30/30/40 plan has also been popular recently. This includes lots of red meat, eggs, all dairy products, poultry, white bread and sugar. It is recommended you eat a full 30% fat especially saturated animal fat. Since the ideal includes only 10% of vegetable oils this is obviously a high fat diet. It also recommended eating 30% protein, which is at least twice what you need. One reason this has become popular is that some movie stars hyped it. Now, that's a great reason to follow such a regimen! The theory is that 30% fat and 30% protein will keep your insulin and glucose at proper levels for optimal blood sugar metabolism. It has been clinically proven very conclusively that eating too much fat and protein especially from animal sources is as much a cause of blood sugar dysmetabolism as is our intake of various simple sugars. It has equally been proven the best way to maintain optimum blood sugar levels is by eating complex whole carbohydrates. This is obviously a very unhealthy diet with three times the fat and twice the protein you need. The claims are made that you will achieve "superhealth", maintain lower insulin levels, lose fat, gain lean muscle mass, have more energy, lower cholesterol and better mental focus. Good luck.

There is even a "breathitarian" diet where you only eat raw fruits and nuts as they fall off the tree naturally and you never kill or hurt anything. You eat nothing but fruit and nuts and eventually try to become so "spiritual" that you need no physical food at all and live off of "prana" or cosmic energy. This is patently ridiculous, but they do have a point here. Essentially nothing in this universe exists except "sat/chit/ananda" which is consciousness, energy and bliss. Food is nothing but manifested energy and, in theory, if you were enlightened you would simply absorb ever-present prana and not need physical food. The physical world is rather different for us regular people unfortunately.

You are welcome to be a pure vegetarian or vegan, which simply means you eat no seafood. If you feel that you should not eat any animal food whatsoever, macrobioitcs is a perfect diet for you. So called "lacto-ovo vegetarians" eat eggs, milk and dairy products. Obviously eggs and milk aren't vegetables and it is rather silly to call yourself a vegetarian when you eat them. Eggs, milk and dairy are among the top ten allergenic foods known and you could never be healthy eating this way. Many vegetarians and vegans are "ethical" by nature and choose not to harm or exploit any animal life including honey from bees or casein in soy cheese. This is to be respected certainly. Unfortunately such people often eat refined foods, junk foods, tropical and Nightshade foods and are outright sugar addicts. Many of them admit they are not eating for health, but only out of compassion for animals. Macrobiotics is a wonderful opportunity for people who want to be pure vegetarians to express their compassion while eating healthful, balanced and nutritious food.

One of the most popular series of diet books was written by a television actress who got breast cancer from following her own advice. Nevertheless, many women still follow her advice!

The Pritikin diet has a lot going for it, but needs to deal with Nightshade vegetables, tropical foods and dairy products. The Ornish diet is a very good, low fat diet but does include Nightshade vegetables and tropical foods; he has dropped dairy products. The McDougall diet is pure vegetarian but also includes Nightshades and tropical foods. The Physician's Committee for Responsible Medicine is a very unusual group of doctors that, not surprisingly includes Neal Barnard and Dean Ornish and advocate a good basic way of eating.

Chapter 9: Natural Hormone Balance

When macrobiotics was introduced to America natural hormones were basically just not available. Doctors rarely — and still don't — test anyone for their hormone levels and it was prohibitively expensive to do so. Scientists were well aware of the importance of the entire endocrine system, but not doctors nor the general public. Technology in the 1990's finally produced supplements of most all the basic hormones inexpensively, and this became an important part of life extension. People who eat well, exercise and live a healthy lifestyle certainly have better hormone profiles than those who don't. However, this doesn't make up for the decline in our "good" hormones and rise of our "bad" hormones as we age. We are going to discuss progesterone, estradiol, estrone, estriol, DHEA, melatonin, testosterone, androstenedione, pregnenolone, cortisol, thyroid and growth hormone, as these are the basic ones we can practically deal with. Surprisingly men and women both have exactly the same hormones, only in different amounts. Women have testosterone and androstenedione and men have prolactin, LH and FSH. The chapter on Home Hormone Testing will tell you how to test these at home using saliva samples without a doctor.

Progesterone is not a feminizing hormone, but rather the antagonist to the estrogens in our bodies, balancing them. Women have been given unnatural oral progesterone analogs (chemical relatives) called "progestins" instead of real, bioidentical progesterone. Men have not been told how important progesterone is for their metabolism and how it protects them from rising estrogen levels as they age. Women with PMS, menstrual irregularities, menopause, osteoporosis, arthritis and other problems can often benefit greatly from transdermal progesterone supplementation. Men over 40 can benefit from using very small amounts of natural progesterone especially to protect them from the current epidemic of prostate disorders. Buy a good two-ounce jar of transdermal cream with 800 to 1000 mg of real USP natural progesterone. Women can read my book "No More Horse Estrogen!" as well as many other books on natural progesterone by John Lee and other authors. Men can read my book "The Natural Prostate Cure". Avoid any products with the word "yam" or "wild yam" on the label as this is called "yam scam" in the trade. Yam (Dioscorea species) extract is used in laboratories as the raw material for conversion to progesterone, but this is NOT a precursor in the body. Progesterone is extremely safe and non-toxic and has many proven benefits.

There is no such thing as "**estrogen**" per se and it is a convenient term that refers to the group of two-dozen or so estrogens. Estradiol is the strongest, estrone second and estriol very mild in comparison. Humans have 80 to 90% estriol and 5 to 10% each of estrone and estradiol. Women who go through menopause are rarely low in estrogen, contrary to the popular wisdom, and giving them estradiol and estrone supplements — especially from horses — only makes them worse, not better. Breast, uterine and ovarian cancers are all basically caused by excessive unopposed (by progesterone) levels of estrogens. American women are generally plagued by excessive levels of estradiol and estrone from overeating, not exercising, consuming almost half their calories from fats, drinking alcohol, and other causes.

Estriol is the "forgotten estrogen" even though it comprises 80 to 90% of human estrogen and is not even manufactured in the U.S. You must obtain a transdermal cream from a compounding pharmacist, if you can find a doctor who is even familiar with using it. If, in fact a woman, tests low in estradiol or estrone she can take real, natural hormones in the amounts she needs, but this not the practice. Doctors who hand out estrogens rarely test the blood levels before prescribing them. Men over 50 have higher estrogen levels than their menopausal wives! This is a frightening fact and a major reason that men have hormonal imbalance as they age. The only realistic way to lower excessive estrogen levels is to eat a low fat diet, exercise, don't drink alcohol and take the supplement DIM (discussed in the supplement chapter). One third of American women consent to being castrated by having their uterus surgically removed (the ovaries die even if not taken out) at an average age of only 35. They must test all their hormone levels after undergoing this procedure.

DHEA is a very powerful hormone and the levels fall after the age of 40. By that age most people have already fallen about 50%. Never, never take DHEA without first testing your level to see if you are deficient. The ideal is always YOUTHFUL levels. Some people naturally have excessive levels of DHEA, which is a pathological state especially in women. If you are deficient men can take about 25 mg and retest their levels after about six months. Women may only need 10 to 20 mg and should also retest after about six months. There are several good books on the benefits of DHEA supplementation, and the scientific literature has literally thousands of studies to prove this; more benefits are discovered every month.

Melatonin is the most underrated of all hormones. The media tells you this is merely for better sleep and jet lag! Melatonin is critical to longevity, how strong your immunity is and how prone you are to getting such diseases as cancer. Good books have been written on melatonin such as "Your Body's Natural Wonder Drug", "Melatonin Miracle", "Melatonin: The Anti-Aging Hormone", "ABC's of Hormones" and "Stay Young the Melatonin Way". The most impressive use is with cancer patients choosing a holistic program of diet, supplements and balancing their other hormones. Melatonin falls from the time we leave our teenage years and keeps falling until we have almost none left by the age of 70. The most important benefit is influencing how long we live since this regulates the aging clock in our bodies. Mice simply given melatonin in their drinking water lived one third longer than control mice. Imagine theoretically living to 100 rather than just 75 by taking two dollars worth of melatonin every month. It is important to take melatonin only at night, as we do not produce this during the day. Three milligrams is a good general dose and you can only test this by itself at 3:00 AM in the morning with a saliva test unless you know a medical doctor who has office hours at that time. This is extremely safe without any known side effects and scientists cannot even find an LD50 (lethal dose in 50% of test animals) for it. There is no such thing as naturally excessive melatonin levels, but it would be very unwise to go over the youthful levels you had in your twenties.

Testosterone is important for both men and women although men have about ten times more of it. Women can have naturally excessive levels as they produce it in very different ways. Men cannot have naturally excessive levels. Testosterone falls in men after the age of 40 and most men are deficient by the age of 50. This level can be raised to the youthful male levels you had in your 20's. You can use oral androstenedione tablets or natural transdermal testosterone cream. It is important you never, never use unnatural oral testosterone salts such as enanthates and propionates. If women are deficient they must use very small doses (like 2 or 3 mg a day) of natural transdermal testosterone cream, since they have very little testosterone compared with men. They can also try 10 to 20 mg of androstenedione since they convert this less efficiently to testosterone than men do. Men who are deficient can use natural testosterone cream in about 15-20 mg a day amounts or use 50 mg tablets of androstenedione. If a man is using 3% natural testosterone cream he would use a half gram a day to get 15 mg. If you want stronger doses use a 5% cream.

Pregnenolone is the "grandparent" hormone since it produces all the other sex hormones ultimately, but it is also the "forgotten" hormone as it has been studied so sparsely. It is incomprehensible why this basic hormone has been ignored since it was discovered. We do know that it is the most important of all brain hormones and very vital to cognition, memory, clear thought processes and general mental ability. Fortunately there is finally a saliva hormone test available for $35, as a blood test is currently about $150 plus the office visit. Both men and women start losing pregnenolone about the age of 35. Men can try 50 mg daily and women also 50 mg but only four times weekly, retest after about six months and adjust your dosage accordingly.

Cortisol is the "stress hormone", and low cortisol is the ideal, while high cortisol generally indicates too much stress. Therefore there are no cortisol supplements to raise your levels. To lower excessive cortisol is difficult as this is usually due to the way one lives. You cannot tell people to simply walk away from a bad marriage, change their profession, give their children away, escape from lifetime poverty or whatever else is upsetting them. Exercise, meditation, sports, hobbies, getting a pet and other such things can lower our cortisol levels. It is said that having high DHEA and low cortisol is a good indication of long life. The best way to test cortisol is to do an all day saliva test since it would be difficult to get an all day blood test. This gives you a better picture of your cortisol secretion, rather than just test it early in the morning at 8:00 or 9:00.

The **thyroid** surprisingly has been neglected in life extension circles and there is no reason for this. Our thyroids secrete two hormones; T3 (triiodothyridine) and T4 (L-thyroxine). About 20% of that is T3 (which is four times stronger than T4) and about 80% is T4. You can get blood or saliva tests but these don't always tell you as much as you would expect since there is such a wide range of values. You can be thyroid excessive (hyperthyroidism) or deficient (hypothyroidism). It is best to go by symptoms as well as blood or saliva levels. Fortunately bioidentical versions of both hormones are easily and inexpensively available. If you are shown to be low in T4 you generally take 25 mcg to 100 mcg to raise your level. If you are shown to be low in T3 you generally take one fourth as much T3 as your would T4 since it is four times stronger. Always test and supplements these SEPARATELY. Most doctors have very little knowledge of this, don't even prescribe T3 and go only by lab results rather than actual known hypothyroid symptoms. T

There are also dried animal thyroid powders which contain both T3 and T4 you can choose, but these are no more natural than the real pharmaceutical hormones and you probably do not need both hormones at all. We need a lot more study and a lot more education in medical schools about thyroid function, symptoms, testing and supplementation. Another way to determine if you are excessive or deficient is to take your temperature every morning for one month. A doctor named Broda Barnes did a lot of work in this area years ago and his books are still available in libraries. It is a much more difficult problem if you have hyperthyroidism as it is very hard to slow the thyroid down except by harmful surgery, dangerous drugs and outright radiation that destroys thyroid tissue. Lifestyle and natural health practices are the real answer.

Lastly we will discuss **growth hormone** (GH). Our growth hormone levels fall from the time we are young and continue to fall until they are extremely low by the age of seventy or so. Only in rare cases of agromely do we see excessive GH levels. You can get great benefits from raising your growth hormone levels if you find that they test low. Currently you cannot get saliva tests for this and the conventional wisdom that IGF-1 (which can easily be saliva tested) parallels growth hormone levels is not true no matter how widespread this misinformation is. You must see a doctor and get a serum test for actual hGH (human growth hormone). The only way to raise your level is by injecting expensive rhGH (recombinant) at least twice a week at a current cost of $300 or more monthly. You can use air injector pens that diabetics use rather than hypodermic needles. No matter what you hear there are NO oral supplements to raise your growth hormone levels. You will see and hear endless ads promising you their supplement is "clinically proven" to work, but none of these have any value at all. You will see some very convincing advertising telling you about oral growth hormone "secretagogues" but none of it is true. In my estimation, none of them work! Period. You will probably need about 30 IU (which is 10 mg) per month of prescription rhGH. You must balance all your other basic hormones to get any real effects out of this.

Our endocrine system is a harmonious balance and the hormones all work together in concert. Raising one deficient hormone and ignoring the others has very little effect on us. Cow (bovine) and pig (porcine) growth hormones are very inexpensive, yet cost no more to produce than the human type. This proves pharmaceutical companies could offer hGH for $100 a month and still make a good profit, but they are unwilling to do so. There are oral and nasal spray secretagogues that will be available within the next five or ten years, but they will be very expensive, sold only by prescription and simply more convenient to use. The most notable of these is hexarelin, which has been proven safe and effective for decades in humans of all ages including GH deficient children, yet is still not available on the market. Many other such substances that may raise our growth hormone levels are constantly being researched and developed. Meanwhile you can take one gram of the common amino acid L-glutamine twice a day to substantially and temporarily spike your GH levels.

Chapter 10: Home Hormone Testing

Thirty years ago the only way to test your hormone levels was to go to a specialist and order very expensive blood tests. Almost no one did this unless they had an unusual disease and were under the care of an endocrinologist. Even then only a very few hormones would be tested. Now most doctors can easily test your basic hormones for about $100 each. Unfortunately most doctors are completely ignorant of this and have no idea at all what to test for or what the results mean. Most doctors don't even know that most of our sex hormones are bound with sex hormone binding globulin (SHBG) and are completely unavailable biologically. This is why, for example they will test your bound testosterone, your free testosterone and then calculate a bound/free ratio — as if all this has some great esoteric meaning. The bound hormone levels are basically meaningless while the unbound, free levels are critical to every facet of our health and wellbeing.

The words "melatonin", "estriol", "pregnenolone", "DHEA", "androstenedione" and other such common hormones just are not in the vocabulary of medical doctors generally. If they can't sell you an expensive prescription for it, they aren't interested in it.

There is a much easier, cheaper and less invasive way to do this at home with a simple saliva sample. For decades clinics have used saliva instead of blood serum to test hormone levels. One of the greatest technological breakthroughs of the last decade has been to simplify and improve these saliva tests so they can be used by people at home, without needing an expensive office visit to a medical doctor. Several major labs now do saliva testing for a wide range of hormones and every year the list of what they can test for grows longer. The World Health Organization approved this for field testing in Third World countries years ago. You simply purchase a saliva kit, spit in a plastic tube and mail it in to the laboratory. Sophisticated RIA (radioimmunoassay) testing accurately determines your hormone levels down to the picogram (billionth of a gram). You get a chart or table to show you the reference values for your age and sex; all this for about $25 to $30 a hormone.

Listed below are five prominent labs. You can also search the Internet under "saliva hormone testing".

Aeron Life Cycle Labs
(now sold thru Jason Products)
8469 Warner Drive
Culver City, CA   90232
(800) 527-6605 toll free

Great Smokies Diagnostics
(aka Body Balance)
18-A Regent Park Blvd.
Asheville, NC   28806
(888) 891-3061 toll free

ZRT Labs
1815 N.W. 169th Place #3090
Beaverton, OR   97006
(503) 466-2445
www.salivatest.com

Pharmasan
375 280th Street
Osceola, WI   54020
(888) 342-7272
www.pharmasan.com

Life-Flo Health Care Products
11202 North 24th Avenue
Phoenix, AZ   85029
(888) 999-7440
  www.life-flo.com

Chapter 11: Natural Supplements

When macrobiotics was introduced in this country there were not a lot of supplements available besides the usual vitamins and minerals. Understandably this way of eating stresses that you get your nutrition from whole foods and not from vitamin and mineral pills. This is very correct as far as it goes. Eating whole natural foods does provide you with all the nutrition you need, and you should never look to compensate a poor diet with vitamin and mineral supplements. Most people get their education on supplements from advertisers and promoters and get very misled most of the time, ending up with supplements that are either useless or actually deleterious. In the last three decades tremendous discoveries have been made in the area of life extension and natural health. Many medical journals now regularly include studies on natural diet and supplements. Using this scientific technology in a sensible and holistic way will now allow us to heal illnesses faster, have stronger immunity, feel better, prevent illnesses and live longer than just relying on the food we eat to be well. The simplistic idea of not using supplements just doesn't stand up at all to the light of reason or science. Let's discuss some of the natural supplements that we can use.

Vitamin E is plentiful in whole grains and you only need about 30 IU a day. People commonly exhibit deficiencies since so few Americans eat whole grains. Taking a supplement of 400 IU has been shown to have very strong benefits especially for the cardiovascular system. A good type to take is the mixed tocopherols instead of the usual alpha tocopherol alone. You can also consider the new tocotrionols. The research on vitamin E goes back decades and is well established.

Glutathione along with S.O.D. (super oxide dismutase) are the two most important antioxidant enzymes in our bodies. Taking glutathione per sé is surprisingly not very effective in raising your levels. Taking NAC (N-acetyl cysteine) 600 mg a day is a much more effective way to do this. Unfortunately oral S.O.D. is ineffective, nasal sprays are considered a prescription drug, and so far no pharmaceutical company is interested in offering them. Few doctors are willing to give injections of S.O.D. even though the proven benefits are most effective since they aren't even aware of it. In the future you'll see more nasal and injectable S.O.D. products as the evidence becomes greater.

Phosphatidyl serine or "PS" is an important chemical in our brains that has been shown to be an important supplement in keeping our brains functioning well as we age. You need 100 mg a day and this is a little pricey but well worth it. PS has only become available in the last few years at a reasonable price through improved technology with research that is very impressive. It is now extracted from soybeans rather than cow brains.

While we're talking about phosphatidyl serine you should know that common soy lecithin is phosphatidyl choline. **Lecithin** is also an important supplement for good arterial health as well as brain function. You can take a 1,200 mg softgel every day. Lecithin has been known about for decades and is also extracted from soybeans.

Recently the amino acid **acetyl-L-carnitine** has become available inexpensively and studies prove the value of taking this for brain metabolism, memory, avoiding senility and Alzheimers, and general cognition. This is not expensive and 500 mg a day should be enough for you or 1,000 mg over the age of 60 or in illness.

You have probably never heard of **beta-sitosterols** even though they exist in literally every vegetable you eat. This is an important supplement for both men and women and you should find a brand with about 300 mg of mixed beta-sitosterols (campesterol, stigmasterol, brassicasterol) This is good for cholesterol metabolism and has shown preventative power in cancers especially of the prostate, breast and colon. Vegetarians get far more plant sterols in their diets than carnivores and omnivores. This is an excellent supplement to help prevent the plague of prostate and breast disease generally. It is the active ingredient in saw palmetto — which is useless because of its insignificant sterol content even in the extracts.

It is important to take a good brand of **acidophilus** with 3 billion or more units and keep it refrigerated. Buy only reputable brands like Jarrow, PB-8, American Health, DDS, Puritan's Pride, Bio-Kaps and others. Try and buy it refrigerated. There is a stable spore form of acidophilus called lactospore you can take along with this that doesn't need refrigeration. Along with the acidophilus and lactospore, I recommend taking one or two 750 mg capsules of FOS (fructo-oligosaccharides) otherwise known as inulin. This is an indigestible sugar that feeds the good bacteria in your colon, but not the bad bacteria. It is important to keep your intestines strong and well balanced as the intestines of Americans are generally in terrible shape due to too many calories, too much fat, and too many toxins like excessive sweeteners, coffee and alcohol. These three supplements taken together along with the next one will do wonders for your intestinal health.

Another way to improve your intestinal health and help your growth hormone levels as well is the inexpensive amino acid **L-glutamine**. Taking a gram of this in the morning and a gram before bed will do a lot for your intestines while spiking your growth hormone levels. This does not permanently raise your growth hormone level all day but does raise them for about two hours. Surgeons are actually giving patients L-glutamine after intestinal surgery to help them heal faster.

Flax oil is a much better source of omega-3 fatty acids than fish liver oil for a variety of reasons. Try to purchase your flax oil refrigerated and keep it refrigerated. We eat far too many omega-6 fatty acids and far too few omega-3s as there are so few good food sources of omega-3'. Valuable lignans are contained in flax oil and this is less susceptible to oxidation than fish liver oils. This is the best source of omega-3 fatty acids known and it is very difficult to get omega-3s even on a macrobiotic diet. Taking a one gram softgel every day will go far to balance the ratio of omega-6 to omega-3 fatty acids in your system.

If you are concerned about arthritis be sure to take **glucosamine sulfate**, but don't fall for the chondroitin promotion. (The chondroitin molecule is too large to pass thru our intestinal walls.) Glucosamine is an important building block in our joints and cartilage but taking this by itself is not enough. This needs co-factors such as vitamins D, E and K as well as sufficient minerals and all trace elements. Vitamin D, for example, does not exist in our food, but is made by our skin on exposure to sunlight. If you live in the southern U.S. and spend time outdoors you may not need this. If you live in the northern U.S. or spend most all your time indoors it would be a good idea to take 400 IU a day or 800 IU if you are elderly or ill. Vitamin K is the "forgotten vitamin" and you can take 80 mcg (that's micrograms) a day if you are not taking a multivitamin that contains this much.

The most powerful immune stimulant known to science is not exotic, outrageously priced bioengineered interferon alpha, but rather a simple extract of yeast and mushrooms (1,3/1,6 configuration) or oats and barley (1,3/1,4 configuration) called **beta glucan**. This has been known for decades, but technology has not been able to inexpensively extract it until about the year 2000. Right now the yeast-derived beta glucan is the strongest and least expensive, and you can take 200 mg a day or 400 mg if you are elderly or ill. The yeast proteins are nearly all removed in the processing so you don't need to worry about yeast allergies. Please read my book "What Is Beta Glucan?" (Safe Goods Publishing), to learn about its proven benefits. Don't take the expensive maitake mushroom extract or other preparations as they have very little beta glucan in them.

It is unrealistic to think that you are going to eat enough soy foods like soybeans, tofu, tempeh, etc. to get any realistic amount of isoflavones in your diet. Drinking a single glass of soymilk daily will add more than 43,000 unnecessary calories a year to your diet. Taking a 40 mg **soy isoflavone supplement** is a practical way to get the valuable benefits of the daidzein and genestein. These are not "phytoestrogens" no matter what you have been told or what you have read — they are unrelated flavones or plant pigments that have nothing whatsoever to do with estrogens. Estrogen of any kind is only found in animals and not in plants; to call isoflavones "phytoestrogens" is totally unscientific and very contrary to fact no matter how many times you read this.

An extract of cruciferous vegetables (broccoli, cauliflower and cabbage) called **indole-3-carbinol** or I3C was discovered to have important anti-cancer properties and to lower and improve the metabolism of estrogens in both men and women. This breaks down to di-indolylmethane or DIM in our digestive system, which is twice as strong — and thus half the price. Find a 200 mg DIM supplement by surfing the Internet as this may be difficult to find in stores or catalogs at fair prices. Pay no more than $20 for 60 capsules of 200 mg each and be sure not to take any less than this as most all brands contain much less.

Coenzyme Q10 or CoQ10 is a very important chemical in our bodies and supplementing this after the age of 40 is very beneficial in many ways. As we age the CoQ10 levels in our organs like our hearts and brains fall severely. The research on this is stunning especially for heart health, insulin regulation, liver function, immunity, anti-cancer activity in general and healthy gums. It is a little pricey, but currently you can find it for less than 50 cents a day and you need 100 mg a day to do any good. If you are ill or elderly take 200 mg. This is a very vital supplement to take and it should be emphasized this should be a part of anyone's supplement program. A strong (0.5% to 1.0%) CoQ10 cream can also be used topically on your face to effectively lessen wrinkles and aging. Nearly all the commercial creams refuse to state how much CoQ10 is contained in them because they contain almost none. Search the Internet for sources and read the label carefully.

Curcumin is an extract of the Indian cooking spice tumeric. Find a supplement with 500 mg of actual curcumoids and do not buy mere tumeric powder. This is a very powerful anti-inflammatory for arthritis and rheumatism, and a powerful anti-oxidant with potent anti-cancer properties. Curcumin is an ancient Ayurvedic remedy known for thousands of years and there are good published clinical studies on this as well.

Quercitin is another natural and very powerful anti-oxidant with clinical research behind it. Quercitin has been known about for a long time but has never been popular despite it's well proven benefits. Find an inexpensive 250 mg to 500 mg supplement.

In all these years of research I have not found any scientific evidence that such supplements as colloidal minerals, coral minerals, colloidal silver, chondroitin (that's right), lycopene, colostrums, noni juice, Tribulus, saw palmetto, Pygeum, homeopathic remedies, spirulina, chorella, PC-SPES, deer antler velvet, oral SOD, maca root or other such promotions have any value at all.

Green tea contains valuable polyphenols with many proven health benefits including anti-cancer activity. Unfortunately green tea is just regular old tea (Thea sinensis) before it is fermented to the common black tea and contains caffeine. The same applies to bancha twig tea. Find a decaffeinated brand of extract as it is not reasonable to think you will drink several cups of decaf green tea every day. Do not drink regular green tea- get the decaf variety.

The macrobiotic diet has been criticized for the low **calcium** intake. Defenders have replied with irrational replies about the calcium content of certain macrobiotic foods. The fact is that calcium is basically found in milk and dairy products and these should not be eaten at all. People in Asia, Africa and other areas who don't eat dairy products and eat far less calcium than we do have much better bone and joint health than Europeans who have the highest calcium intake on earth. If you feel the need to take calcium supplements just take 600 to 800 mg and be sure to take magnesium and boron with it as co-factors.

It can be difficult to get all the **minerals and trace elements** we need no matter how well we eat due to depleted soils among other factors. There are 16 minerals we are known to need, as we seem to get enough potassium, sodium, and phosphorous, which leaves 13 you should supplement. Unfortunately almost every single mineral supplement doesn't contain or has insignificant amounts of magnesium, calcium, boron, vanadium, silicon, iron, selenium, chromium, iodine, molybdenum, zinc, manganese and copper. Others such as tin, cobalt and strontium need more research. Such minerals as silica and vanadium are rarely in any vitamin and mineral supplements in needed quantities. Avoid colloidal minerals as well as coral minerals as they never list the amounts of individual minerals contained, have no advantage over natural mineral salts and are simply another commercial promotion. They contain completely insignificant amounts of the dozens of minerals they claim to contain as well as deadly poisons such as arsenic, cadmium and thallium. Search the internet for a brand that has the proper amounts of all thirteen of these in the amounts you need as nearly every single mineral supplement currently sold is very defective.

Whole grains are an excellent source of **magnesium**. So why consider a magnesium supplement? Because many people react very well to taking a magnesium supplement of about 250 to 500 mg regardless of sufficient dietary intake. For example calcium cannot be absorbed without magnesium and boron present. Women especially seem to benefit from taking this for reproductive health and bone strength among other benefits. Boron is deficient in American soils generally, deficient in our foods and therefore deficient in our bodies. You cannot absorb calcium without magnesium and boron. Besides calcium, magnesium and boron be sure to include the other ten minerals we are known to need.

Aloe vera is an old standard because it works. This is well known for topical use, but taking it internally can be good if you have poor digestion, stomach ulcers, or blood sugar dysmetabolism. It is also claimed to be good for immune enhancement, therefore this can generally be considered a universal supplement. Very concentrated 200:1 powdered extracts in capsules are now sold inexpensively which makes it easier to take than spoonfuls of refrigerated gel. Take 100 mg of a good extract.

Let's talk about **vitamin C**. The macrobiotic diet has been criticized for its low amount of vitamin C. The reality is that the recommended daily allowance is only 60 mg a day and you will get enough eating green and yellow vegetables, as well as local fruit in moderation. Vitamin C is extremely yin and generally the only high source of vitamin C is tropical foods especially tropical fruits and Nightshade plants like tomatoes. Such foods are meant for people living in those hot tropical areas. Foods grown in temperature climates just do not have high levels of vitamin C as they aren't needed. I feel that you do not need a vitamin C supplement and there is really no reason to take one. If you feel for some reason you want one, take no more than 250 mg a day. Never consider taking large doses of this no matter what nonsense you've read about the value of megadoses. I believe that Linus Pauling was wrong and long-term megadoses are very debilitating, keeping your blood acidified. This will only alter the inherent alkalinity of your blood, lower your immunity and make you sick and debilitated in the end. Please remember that people in temperate climates have done just fine on the vitamin C in their local foods for thousand of years before very recently when transportation advances allowed us to ship tropical fruit to the colder climates.

A popular criticism of vegetarian and macrobiotic diets is the lack of **vitamin B-12** since this is only found in animal foods. Therefore supplements of B-12 are recommended especially for children and babies. Do you really think nature is so inept as to forget to put vitamin B-12 into vegetable foods? Or do you think that we're supposed to eat red meat just to get vitamin B-12? Do you really think logical, rational science is more intelligent than the Infinite Forces of the universe? Did you ever notice that all the countless millions of pure vegetarians in the world for thousands of years have never had a problem with this? Such people as strict Hindu vegetarians have lived healthfully for thousands of years never touching a food of animal origin. Doesn't that answer any questions about needing B-12 supplements? We make our own B-12 in our intestines every day and when we eat well we always have enough of it. B-12 supplements are very poorly absorbed and effective nasal sprays are considered a drug. Women should include 400 to 800 mcg of folic acid and 10 mg of B-6.

Chapter 12: Tropicals and Nightshades

The macrobiotic philosophy has always been the only method of eating that warns against Nightshade vegetables, also known as the Solanaciae family botanically. This includes potatoes, tomatoes (botanically a fruit), eggplants and most peppers, belladonna, Jimson weed and tobacco. You can see this family includes delerium inducing, toxic and deadly plants. These vegetables contain harmful glycoalkaloids especially solanine and chaconine. The average American eats enough solanine alone every year to kill a family of four if it was eaten all at once. Why do so few diet authors not understand Nightshade vegetables should be excluded from our diet due to these harmful alkaloids?

Green skinned potatoes are so dangerous they are unsafe to eat because of the very high level of alkaloids. Potato sprouts also contain equally dangerous amounts. Potatoes can range widely in alkaloid content, but about 12 mg per 100g serving is typical. Some varieties contain up to 30 mg per 100g serving. These are dangerous amounts clearly.

Have you noticed all the Caucasian-developed countries seem to live off meat and potatoes? Americans, Canadian, English, Scotch, Welsh, Irish, Germans, Poles, French, Swiss, Austrians, Australians and New Zealanders all love potatoes and use them as a major staple in their diet. Americans are estimated to eat over 60 kg a year, which comes to about 170 grams per day. Mashed potatoes, baked potatoes, the ubiquitous French fry, hash browns, potato pancakes, potato chips, and potato salad. Why this love affair with a mere tuber other than the fact it is inexpensive, easy to grow and very versatile? The Asian countries did not eat potatoes until very recently and still do not embrace them.

The tomato for centuries was considered an ornamental plant unfit to eat. We should have retained that native wisdom and kept them for decoration. It is only recently that Americans started to eat large amounts of tomatoes and tomato products especially canned ones. In addition to solanine the tomato also contains the glycoalkaloid tomatine, which has similar toxic effects. This is not native to America and was introduced over two hundred years ago. Tomatoes are one of the top ten known allergenic foods. Many people break out if they eat them, yet millions of tons are eaten every year in ketchup, pasta sauce, pizza and other foods.

Southern Italy is the major country to make a cult of the tomato. Nearly all natural-diet authors include tomatoes as a regular staple and just don't understand how toxic the Solanum vegetables are. If you ate just one tomato a day for a year the solanine in them would actually kill an entire family if ingested all at once.

Eggplants (Solanun melongena) are just not very popular and never have been fortunately. The amount of solanine varies but typically is about 8 mg per 100 g serving ranging from about 6 to 11 mg. Avoid eating eggplants.

Peppers (Capsicum family) including bell peppers are very popular in America but contain similar amounts of solanine of about 8 mg per 100g serving. They can only be used occasionally and in small amounts. This does not include black pepper but that should be avoided for other reasons.

One major reason for the epidemic of arthritis and rheumatism we have is our intake of solanine alkaloids. These do accumulate in our tissues over time. Many studies have shown the effect of Nightshade vegetables on joint inflammation in both lab animals and humans. Many people have gotten dramatic relief from taking these out of their diet completely. A very good article was in the Journal of Neurological and Orthopedic Medical Surgery in 1993 (vol. 12, p. 227-31) with a long list of references.

Solanine poisoning has effects we still do not know about, but the known ones include nausea, diarrhea, abdominal cramps, coma, fever, headache, weak pulse, delerium, rapid breathing and hallucinations. There have been recorded incidents of mass poisoning in Europe earlier in this century when poor people ate large amounts of potatoes, as they had no other food to eat.

Macrobiotic philosophy was about the only system of eating to tell people in temperate climates not to eat tropical foods. Why haven't the other diet authors understood this rather obvious fact? Foods grown in tropical areas are extremely yin to balance their extremely yang environment. Nature has a pattern here, and the foods that grow in hot, tropical climates like mangos, bananas, citrus fruit, avocados, and coconuts are meant for the indigenous peoples in those areas to adapt to such a climate. If you would feed an Eskimo such foods they would sicken and quickly die. Or if you fed someone in Southern India nothing but fish, whale and seal meat and fat they would also sicken and die quickly.

The situation gets much more confusing when people of European descent move to tropical areas to live rather than merely visit. Or when people from Africa, the Philippines or Southern India move to temperate climates to make their home. All these people are going against the order of the universe and not harmonizing their genetics with their environment. Take for example, people of African descent; in Africa there really is very little typical western disease like colon cancer, breast cancer, lung cancer, prostate cancer, diabetes, high blood pressure, atherosclerosis and heart attack. African men and women who live in America and Europe have stratospheric rates of all these diseases from an environment and diet not meant for their genetics. The same is true for Europeans who move to tropical climates. There are no easy answers for these people. Our bodies are a microcosm of the universe and we also are microcosms of the environment we live in.

The point is to eat foods that grow in temperate climates and avoid foods that grow in tropical climates. Alexis Carrel in his book, "Man, the Unknown" writes, "Man is literally made from the dust of the earth. For this reason, his physiological and mental activities are profoundly influenced by the geological constitution of the country where he lives, by the nature of the animals and plants he eats." We are healthier, stronger and in tune with the universal laws when we eat the food in our environment that was given to us by Nature to be appropriate. The United States in recent years has a very high consumption of various citrus fruits and citrus juice for example. Orange juice for breakfast is an American tradition. Citrus fruits are plentiful, inexpensive and widely consumed — and contribute very much to the bad health of our country. This is especially true when they are eaten in the winter, which is very yin.

Have you ever noticed that vitamin C is basically only found in any quantity in tropical fruits (also in the Nightshade fruit tomatoes) like mangoes, papayas, citrus fruits and the like? These fruits are meant for the indigenous peoples of hot tropical areas, as they need more vitamin C than we do. There is very sufficient vitamin C in the fresh green and yellow vegetables we eat in temperature climates, so we have no need at all to eat tropical fruits or take vitamin C supplements. In fact this can be counterproductive as this is a very yin vitamin and tends to acidify our normally alkaline blood. Since citrus fruit is very inexpensive and available year round, this has become a staple in American culture. When people have a cold or flu they actually are told to drink more orange and grapefruit juice, which just makes them worse of course.

There is a third group of foods to be cautious of and that is the oxylate group. Most common vegetables contain small amounts of oxalic acid, but the following foods contain higher quantities than other vegetables and should only be eaten occasionally. Oxalic acid binds with minerals especially calcium and iron to form urinary stones. Vegetables such as Swiss chard, spinach, sorrel, amaranth, rhubarb, beet leaves, parsley, purslane, chives and cassava root contain high amounts of oxalic acid that contribute to poor health if eaten regularly. These foods can be eaten occasionally in small amounts though.

Avocados are a popular fruit because of the very high (78%) fat content. One cup of California avocado contains a whopping 407 calories, four fifths of which are from fat (36 grams of fat). Most vegetarian eat tropical fruits such as avocados regularly, and this is one reason vegetarianism as practiced does not work very well; there is no understanding of the Order of the Universe. You' find most vegetarians tend to be sugar addicts and eat large amounts of sweet tropical fruits such as mangoes and bananas and "natural" sweeteners such as honey thinking these are good for them. Sugar is sugar is sugar and all simple mono- and disaccharides have the same basic deleterious effects on us when eaten in any quantity.

Chapter 13: Exercise

*The sovereign invigorator of the body is
exercise, and of all the exercises walking is the best.*
– Thomas Jefferson

Surprisingly traditional macrobiotics did not stress exercise. People in poor Third World countries usually have to do manual labor and walk many miles a day just to stay alive. In the developed countries of the world people actually have to go to swimming pools, gymnasiums and health clubs, tennis courts and other places to get exercise. Unfortunately most people in America just don't bother. Even if you enjoy skiing, tennis, soccer, basketball, softball and other sports you just aren't going to get regular year round workouts from these kinds of activities. You can choose aerobic exercise (the kind that makes you pant) or resistance exercise (weight training) or, ideally, a combination of both. Many runners, for example, have poor upper body strength while many weight trainers have poor aerobic capacity. Most people have jobs, children and endless responsibilities that leave little time or energy for exercise even if it is just walking the dog every night. Yet a third type of exercise is internal and expressed in such disciplines as aikido, tai chi, and chi gong, which are meditative and spiritual in nature.

The best overall exercise is simply walking briskly at a pace of about four miles an hour. Just a half-hour walk each day will keep you in shape, but a whole hour would be ideal. Walking will do wonders for you physically as well as mentally. A daily walk will lower your blood pressure, help relieve stress, suppress appetite, help you lose weight beyond merely burning calories, circulate your blood and improve blood parameters, stimulate digestion, relax you, help you sleep better, improve your appearance, prevent coronary heart disease, lower your cholesterol and gives you a wonderful time to reflect on your life and deal with your everyday situations. The other aerobic exercise is jogging, but most people simply don't enjoy this. Jogging can have side effects such as shin splints, bone spurs, runner's knee (inflammation), foot stress mini-fractures and swelling of the Achille's tendon; so be careful if you choose this.

Resistance exercise or weight training is for both men and women, especially ones over the age of 30. Women gain strength and tone while men gain strength and size. Strength training raises your level of "beta-endorphins" which make you feel good all the time, diminishes or eliminates mood swings and prevents or stops depression. Doing 50 sets of weights twice a week is enough to keep anyone in good shape and this can be done in a mere half hour with "circuit training". People who really want to be in top shape can do 50 sets three times a week. Circuit training is just doing one exercise after another with only about fifteen seconds of resting between sets. You can learn to do 50 sets in just 15 minutes this way. Circuit training is also aerobic.

The epidemic of osteoporosis especially among women also is a factor for men. It is very difficult to rebuild bone once it is lost no matter how good your diet, supplement program and hormone profile. A far easier method to prevent osteoporosis includes resistance exercise to stress your bones and tell them to be stronger. This is one reason poor people in Third World countries have much stronger bones and less bone and joint disease — they have to work hard physically and put stress on their bones all throughout their lives.

Professional athletes such as football and baseball and basketball players actually live shorter lives, and suffer from more ills than most of us? One reason is they only stay conditioned for a short period in their life and this is not a long-term lifestyle. Another reason is most of them eat high protein, high fat, high sugar diets based on meat, poultry, eggs and dairy products. This shows that exercise must be a lifelong commitment especially in our latter years.

You can never be slim, trim, fit, feel good and stay youthful all your life without some kind of regular exercise. Admittedly we live in a technological society where most of us work with our minds rather than our hands. Find the kind of exercise you enjoy and stay with it the rest of your life. Physical fitness is priceless and a cornerstone of good health.

Chapter 14: Fats and Oils

It is important that you eat a low fat diet for many reasons. There are only three sources of calories — carbohydrates at 5 calories per gram, proteins at 5 calories and fats at 9 calories. Fats of all kinds contain almost twice the calories of carbohydrates or proteins. Since you will not be eating red meat, poultry, eggs, milk or dairy products, it is really quite easy to keep your fat calorie intake down to 10 or 15 per cent. 20 per cent is the very maximum and there is no reason to eat that much. Please do not think that vegetables oils are somehow "good for you", as unsaturated vegetable oils are simply less harmful than saturated animal fats. Clinical studies have shown that sometimes vegetable oils can promote cancer cell growth every bit as well as the saturated fats. Saturated fats are only found in animal foods. Palm and coconut oils are actually not saturated at all since they are liquid in the hot tropical areas they are native to. The fats in fish and seafood are not harmful in moderation and do not raise your cholesterol and triglyceride levels.

You actually do not need any vegetable oil in your kitchen and many native peoples simply do not use this in their food preparation. You can use oils in moderation for stir-frying, baking, salad dressing and other limited uses. What oils are good for general use? All the oils you see in the grocery store are generally heavily refined and heated to high temperatures and filtered to make them clear and more appealing visually. Virgin olive oil is one of the only exceptions. The cold pressed oils in the natural food store can be quite expensive. You are getting very little nutrition from oil anyway, so in this sense it just doesn't matter very much. Also any solvents that are used to extract oil are boiled off basically. It is your choice whether to buy grocery store oils or natural food store oils, but in either case, use as little as possible.

Corn oil is a fine choice especially since it comes from grain. Safflower and sunflower oils are both good choices. Sesame oil is good but just too expensive for general use. Toasted sesame or "dark sesame" oil is an excellent condiment for Asian dishes. Olive oil is a good choice but it is not "good for you" no matter what you have read. Soy oil does not taste good unless it has been very heavily refined. Peanut oil comes from one of the top ten allergenic foods and is not a good choice at all.

Cottonseed oil is purely a commercial byproduct of the cotton industry and was never meant for human consumption. This is a favorite oil for hydrogenation since it is the least expensive edible oil. Walnut, avocado, pumpkin seed, almond and other gourmet oils make nice specialty oils but are very expensive and have limited use. Avoid anything that has the generic description "vegetable oil" or "vegetable oil blend" as you can count on the fact this is based on cheap cottonseed oil. Palm and coconut oil are tropical foods and should be eaten by tropical people living in their native climates. They are all right for occasional use though.

Canola oil needs a separate mention. The name comes from "Canadian oil" and the source is the rapeseed (Latin for rapa or turnip). This is promoted in the natural foods industry as a healthy oil to use, when it certainly is not. Canola oil by law must contain less than 2% of the toxic erucic acid that is naturally contained in it. For many years rapeseed oil could only be fed to farm animals or used in industrial applications because of the high erucic acid content. This is a major crop in the cold Canadian climate and the farmers genetically engineered this over the years to make it "acceptable" for human use. This was never meant for human consumption and no amount of genetic engineering will make it so. Do not buy or use products with canola oil no matter how promoted they are in the so-called natural foods industry. The fact that the entire natural food industry is promoting this as a healthy choice tells you a lot about the people in it and their real motivations; also their intelligence.

Americans eat the most fat of anyone one earth (except Eskimos who have a very short lifespan and live under the most primitive of conditions). On the average people in America eat an astounding 42% fat calories and most of these are from animal fats. Five times the amount of fats we need. And we wonder why we have such epidemics of cancers, CHD, diabetes and other diseases?

Macrobiotic people have cholesterol levels of about 150, low triglyceride levels and excellent HDL to LDL ratios. Total cholesterol is an excellent predictor of life span. They also have very low cancer rates as you can see by the following charts on breast and prostate cancer. Men with very low fat intake, especially animal fats, rarely get prostate disease of any kind.

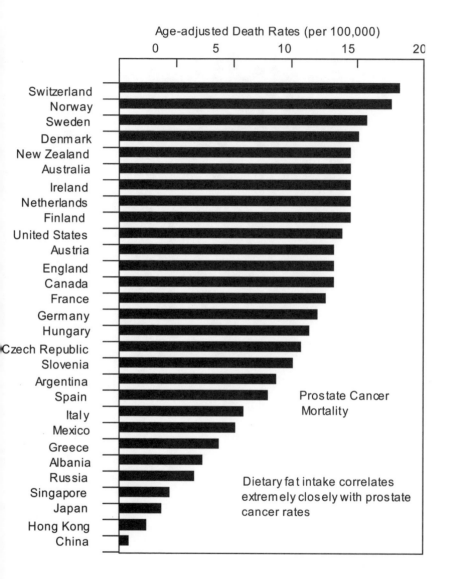

Age-adjusted Death Rates (per 100,000)

Prostate Cancer
Mortality

Dietary fat intake correlates
extremely closely with prostate
cancer rates

65

International Breast Cancer Death Rates Related to Fat Intake

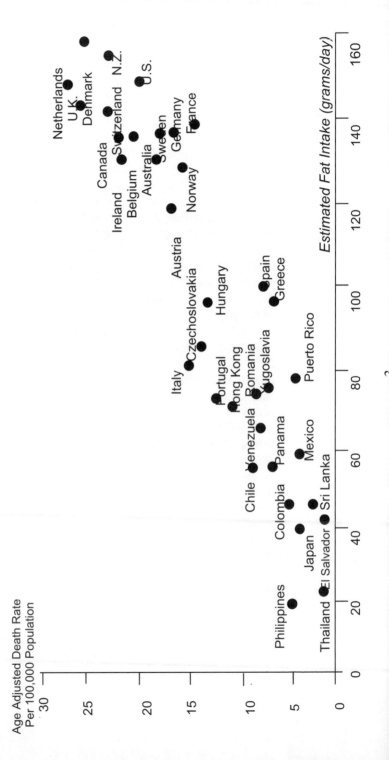

Chapter 15: Curing the Incurable

> *Doctors are men who prescribe medicines of which they know little, to cure diseases of which they know less, to human beings of which they know nothing.*
> - Voltaire

What is it that distinguishes the macrobiotic diet from the countless other diets that are all claimed to be the best for us? What proof is there that eating whole grains, beans and vegetables as our basic foods is really the ideal way of eating? Why should we put any faith in books such as this one? It's very simple...what other way of eating allows one to cure themselves of "incurable" diseases such as various cancers, diabetes, epilepsy, atherosclerosis and other such illnesses that allopathic medicine can only cover up with palliatives? Remember that it is not diet that cures disease, but rather that our bodies cure themselves. Healthy eating allows our own healing powers to cure illness. It is common and everyday in macrobiotic circles to talk about people who have cured different kinds of cancer in less than a year. Or people who were living on insulin to have normal blood sugar levels after two years of eating natural foods in the macrobiotic tradition. Talk to someone who was afflicted with epilepsy and was on brain deadening seizure medication who is now healthy and clear minded after a few years of this lifestyle.

Every year cancer becomes more common, and now one in three people will end up with cancer before they die. There will never be a "cure" for cancer, as the real cure has always been to be in harmony with natural laws. The phony "War on Cancer" has done nothing but waste money on allopathic studies, and the cancer occurrence and survival rates have only worsened. This is neither random nor caused by events beyond our control. Certainly there are genetic and environmental influences, but our diet and lifestyle are the basic causes. Diseases are a wake-up call from Nature to change our direction. This is not a "war" or a "fight" at all as we so often hear. Americans eat twice the calories we need, five times the fat we need, twice the protein we need, 125 pounds of sugars we don't need at all, God knows how much coffee, alcohol and cigarettes, plus an endless variety of refined foods full of chemicals, preservative, additives and colorings. And then we wonder why we have such high rates of disease? Take the time to read some classic books on natural healing. Anthony Satarillo was a medical doctor who was dying of pancreatic cancer and believed only in dogmatic allopathic medicine. He completely turned his view around and cured himself and wrote the book "Recalled by Life".

Milenka Dobic had stage IV ovarian cancer, which had already metastasized into her liver and lymph system. She was only given a few months to live. Milenka had a husband and daughter and was just too young to die. She was ready to go through the usual surgery, radiation and chemotherapy until she met women in her doctor's waiting room who were barely alive after going through this. She saw the living hell they were suffering and felt death would be preferable. Somehow, even in Yugoslavia, she found out about macrobiotics and immediately changed her way of life. She and her family started eating whole grains, beans and vegetables instead of meats, chicken, potatoes, eggs, milk and dairy products. Her health kept improving and within two years she was cancer free. She wanted to share her experience with the world and wrote the book "My Beautiful Life".

Dirk Benedict was a famous, rich and happy actor who got prostate cancer in his thirties and decided he wanted to live rather than be butchered, irradiated and poisoned. In less than a year he was well and wrote "Confessions of a Kamikaze Cowboy". He is now in his fifties, alive, youthful, charismatic, creative, and the father of two handsome sons.

Elaine Nussbaum was a Jewish housewife who thought the sun rose and set on medical doctors. She let them literally destroy her when she got cancer until she was at the brink of death. She refused to die and got well within two years and wrote "Recovery from Cancer". She was diagnosed with advanced uterine cancer and given twenty radium treatments as well as a radium implant. She then had both her uterus and ovaries removed. Then she went on to chemotherapy. She then got cancer of the spine and both lungs and got ten more radium treatments for a total of thirty exposures. She went on to more chemotherapy and then to antibiotics and numerous blood transfusions as she could no longer stop bleeding. She was taking over three dozen pills a day now. Near death and complete collapse she read "Recalled by Life" and changed the entire course of her life. She started eating macrobiotic food and within two years was cancer free and gaining strength. She went on to live, write her book and become a dietary counselor to others.

There are many thousands of people who have read these books and cured themselves of all manner of "incurable" illnesses and never wrote a book, so you'll never hear of them. I have been fortunate enough to work with men with prostate cancer for years now who just did not want to end up as the living dead. They saw no reason to be technically alive as suffering zombies. They choose to change their lifestyle and the food they ate. Every one of them, who made a sincere attempt to cure themselves, was well within less than a year; there were no failures except the ones who didn't have the faith and judgment to change their lives and went to the medical doctors for their allopathic treatments.

Diabetes is another epidemic and can be cured by taking all sugars out of your diet including fresh fruit, fruit juices, dried fruit and any sweeteners whatsoever. Have you noticed how uncommon diabetes is in Asia generally especially in the countryside? The same is true in the African and Latin countries generally. If you are on oral or injected insulin you can gradually wean yourself from this. In 2003 I promise to write a book, "The Natural Diabetes Cure." Refined grains and high fat intake are other causes of this besides the extreme sugar intake of modern people. With diabetes you cannot fast even for one day. You can keep going for longer and longer periods of time between eating until you can go a full day comfortably without any food and without any side effects. Continue to fast one day a week, but do not do this until you can do it without discomfort.

What "incurable" illness do you have? There is no reason you cannot heal yourself and be well if you truly want to live. There are two reservations that should be mentioned — AIDS and radiation poisoning, since they are both manmade and not natural diseases. AIDS is the product of genetic bioengineering from military laboratories and not from "green monkeys" in Africa. HIV positive people who have adopted a macrobiotic lifestyle went on to live their lives never progressing to AIDS. Once AIDS takes over you can live longer and better, but there is no cure. There is no concentrated radiation anywhere on the face of the earth and this is a product of technology. Nathan Pritikin died of radiation-induced cancer after he received radium treatments when he was younger. He lived a much longer time with a far higher quality of life by following his own advice — the Pritikin Diet — which was very close to macrobiotics. Once exposed to excessive doses of radiation you can only mollify the effects.

Alzheimer's disease is something that can definitely be prevented by a macrobiotic lifestyle, but once it takes hold there is no cure for it either. The emphasis here is that it CAN be prevented and you can be insured and protected against ever coming down with it by following the principles of natural diet, natural supplements and hormone balance. This is an illness that has only occurred in the last two centuries basically and was non-existent before this; Alzheimers is clearly different from common senility. The Journal of the American Medical Association in 1991 (volume 265, page 313) said that Alzheimers had increased a full thirteen times in the last ten years. It has gotten worse since then. It is quite distinct from classic dementia and we have not figured out what has caused this very recent epidemic. Aluminum is indicated but may simply be a symptom rather than a cause.

This is a good place to talk about allergenic foods. I've found that milk and dairy is the number one allergenic food due to the lactose content. The other top allergens are citrus fruit, chocolate, coffee, alcohol, poultry, eggs, strawberries, Nightshade vegetables (potatoes, tomatoes, eggplants and peppers) and peanuts. Any simple sugars including all fruits are bad for people with candida yeast syndrome. Unfortunately a few people are allergic to fish and seafood. It is popular to say that wheat, corn and soy are among the top allergens but this doesn't seem to work that way in the real world. We do not know how to diagnose allergies however and the current tests that claim to do so simply do not work no matter what their assertions. When we are able to diagnose which foods are compatible for each individual a new day will dawn on natural medicine.

Chapter 16: What to Drink

The best drink in the world is pure water. Nothing is more delicious when you're thirsty than good well or spring water. Distilled water is not how Nature produces it, but it is an acceptable drink. If you do not have well water you can buy inexpensive and very effective water filters for your drinking and cooking needs. The inexpensive ceramic filter models work very well.

It is surprising to many people to learn that we should only drink when we are thirsty. We should only drink when we need to drink, when we have a true thirst. We never have a false thirst for water like we have a false thirst for food. Many dietary advocates advise drinking literally quarts of water per day whether you are thirsty or not. Do *not* listen to this. This drink-as-much-as-you-can theory is very harmful — "drink eight glasses a day". The proponents go on the theory you can flush your kidneys out like sewer pipes. Quite the opposite is true in that the more you drink the less efficiently your kidneys operate. Your kidneys are not like the plumbing system in your house. Kidneys filter, absorb and diffuse and thus cannot be overloaded with water they don't want nor need. Drinking when you're not thirsty overworks them so they can't do what they are designed to do. When you drink too much the kidney cells close up so water can barely pass through. The large intestine in desperation feeds water to the bladder to be passed out without removing the toxins from your system. This leaves the toxins in your body.

Have you ever noticed, for example, people who drink a lot of beer or soft drinks? They urinate a lot but they only urinate colorless water basically with very little toxins being removed from the body. Unlike the hunger instinct when we often eat when we're really not hungry, the feeling of thirst is always a true one. We never feel thirsty unless we really need water. ONLY DRINK WHEN THIRSTY and never drink if you are not thirsty. Your urine should never be cloudy, but rather clear with a deep yellow color to show that lots of toxins are contained in it. It is very difficult to drink when you're not thirsty. It goes against our very instincts to drink when we don't need to drink. It is said that men should urinate three times a day and women only twice. There is a point here in that men do urinate more than women, but we definitely should not be passing urine five, six or more times a day. This clearly indicates kidney problems.

Salt intake is most important. Traditional macrobiotics includes too much salt with all the miso, shoyu, gomashio, and pickled vegetables. Salt is necessary and is good for us in small amounts, but avoid high intakes of salt even in summer when you work outside. Excess salt causes edema (water retention), which unbalances and strains the body when all the excess sodium is excreted in the perspiration and urine. Avoid an over consumption of salt or your body will swell up with water to absorb it.

Coffee is a toxin with not only caffeine, but many other alkaloids, oils and chemicals. Coffee is an insidious national addiction currently and very hard to stop. Decaffeinated coffee is half as bad as regular coffee and not acceptable at all. The clinical research proves that drinking coffee regularly is extremely harmful in many ways and predisposes us to many illnesses and weight gain. Yes, coffee is most enjoyable, inexpensive, legal, available everywhere, popular and can actually help you to work harder and work better. The price you pay for all this is simply too high however. Yerba mate and guarana tea are less harmful and habituating, but nonetheless still caffeine analogs. People are understandably looking for energy drinks and these are promoted as "traditional native tonics". The truth is that they are less harmful alternatives to coffee.

Milk was discussed in a previous chapter. Milk is never suitable, even the low fat, non-fat, lactose reduced or when taken with lactase tablets. No adult of any race produces the enzyme lactase after the age of 5 and all people are lactose intolerant. If the lactose simply passed through your system undigested this wouldn't be a problem — but it doesn't. Soymilk has about 120 calories per cup, which adds an impressive 43,000 calories per year to your dietary intake. Beer is full of alcohol and the less alcohol you drink the better your health will be. Non-alcoholic beer at least is a better choice. Soft drinks no matter how "natural" or new age are full of various sweeteners, especially fructose, and all sugars are sugars regardless of their source.

Artificially sweetened drinks are much worse than real sugars and a new artificial sweetener is introduced every few years with endless guarantees of its safety. Every one of these artificial non-caloric sweeteners has eventually been found to be toxic and unsafe. The newest one claims to be, "made from sugar, tastes like sugar". The truth is this is a synthetic laboratory toxin halogenated with chlorine. New sweetener substitutes are always being contrived such as stevia herb and lo han fruit. There's no way around this folks — you have to severely limit sweets, as they are all extremely yin when used regularly. You'll get used to this very soon.

Traditional macrobiotics is also against ice and iced drinks. If you want to put ice in your water or drink it ice cold just sip it slowly as to not shock your stomach. People who gulp ice cold drinks down on a hot day often get a stomach cramp that will drop them to their knees. You just don't need ice in your drinks.

You'll notice when you fast that you hardly drink at all. When you fast you may only drink two cups of water a day. When you eat less and only eat two small meals a day you drink less. When you add very little salt to your food you'll notice you drink very little. When you eat a lot of salty food like sushi dipped in soy sauce you'll notice an inordinate thirst for several hours and then excessive urination to rid yourself of the extra sodium. The body balances itself very well, but we have to be careful not to go to excesses that disturb this equilibrium and use too much energy to maintain balance. Drink pure water as your main drink, drink as little as possible and do not use excess salt, which causes unnecessary thirst and imbalance. Thirst caused from heavy exercise and hard work is beneficial for us as the water is lost through perspiration and toxins are excreted very well through the skin (our largest organ).

Some people will think they are missing nutrients by not drinking fruit juice. As you saw in the "Fruits and Sugars" chapter, fruits and fruit juice have very little and very limited nutrition. There is as much or even more sugar in fruit juices than commercial soft drinks. Fruit juice is just not healthy to drink. A typical can of cola drink contains about 40 grams of sugars, but many fruit juices contain 48 grams or a full 20% *more* than colas. All regular sugars are "natural" and they are all just as harmful in excess. Sugar is sugar is sugar and all simple sugars are harmful in excess. Once you get off your sugar addiction you'll find that undiluted fruit juices are simply too sweet and cloying. If you want to drink a fruit juice occasionally just use one part juice and three parts water.

What about teas? The term "tea" really refers to the traditional tea plant Thea sinensis. Black tea is the fermented green tea leaf that most people drink, including the Chinese and the English — what is sold in tea bags in the grocery store. Green tea is the unfermented leaf the Japanese drink, but this, unfortunately, is full of caffeine. You can buy decaffeinated green tea very easily and this is a good choice. Bancha (kukicha) tea is promoted in traditional macrobiotics as a healthful beverage, but is full of caffeine despite the fact it is comprised of roasted tea plant twigs. There is no doubt that caffeine is a poison. Why would nature give us a drink that is full of caffeine and must be decaffeinated? If this concerns you then don't drink tea at all. The science on the polyphenols and cathechins in green tea is undeniable on the other hand. Here we have no easy answers. Mu tea is promoted in traditional macrobiotics as some kind of traditional panacea, but is simply an overpriced, traditional drink with no real health benefits.

There are many herbal teas available, but most of these contain herbs that may be incompatible with your individual biochemistry. Use ones make from mint, citrus peel, berry leaves, chicory root and other mild ingredients. One answer is to buy herbal tea bags but only use one bag per 1.5 quart (six cups) teapot. To use one tea bag dilutes this down to amounts that are pretty much biologically insignificant yet still very tasty. Drink good water. Drink water with your meals. Keep a bottle of water in your car. Drink water when you eat out or socialize. Drink water when you travel. This is the very best drink for you.

Chapter 17: Everyday Eating

There is just no reason to eat three meals a day. Eating two meals a day makes life much simpler, as Thoreau suggested when he said, "simplify, simplify, simplify." Eating two meals a day makes it far easier to cook, to eat well, to make good food choices, to limit your caloric intake while not being hungry, and to avoid eating out regularly. Ideally a snack in the morning and just one main meal is the best way to live, but it usually takes years to achieve this and still really enjoy yourself.

One important tenet in eating well is to avoid eating out as much as possible. Take your lunch to work definitely. Either eat breakfast at home and skip lunch, or take your own food. Take some food with you when you go out instead of buying it. The best places to eat are generally Asian restaurants — Thai, Korean, Chinese, Japanese and Vietnamese. The white rice they serve is not a problem, as you'll only be doing this occasionally. You'll find that whenever you go out to eat you end up ingesting something you shouldn't and wouldn't be eating at home. Buffets can be quite good with a wide selection of various fresh vegetables and salads. Mexican restaurants usually have vegetarian dishes, but ask that the cheese not be added to them. Indian restaurants have a tradition of vegetarianism, but avoid the dairy products. Latin restaurants such as Cuban usually have a tradition of rice and beans with various vegetables. Vegetarian restaurants are usually only found in larger cities.

This way of eating and drinking should be FUN and not dull, boring, bland or restrictive. When you see the very wide range of healthy, delicious, whole natural grains, beans, green and yellow vegetables, seafood, salads and local fruits that are included you do not feel limited at all. While the Asians in general are the best vegetable cooks, this is only one type of international cuisine. You can modify many Indian, Northern Italian, French, Mexican, Latin, Cuban, Mediterranean, Mideastern and South American recipes so they are in tune with universal principles. Go get some cookbooks from your local library and try some new ideas on how to cook and season the normal foods you already eat in new ways.

What about babies? It is simply unbelievable that less than half the mothers in America nurse their babies by choice. A very few are physically unable to nurse, which speaks about their condition of health and why they are not physically fit to give birth. Babies should be fed human milk, as this is obviously what is meant for them. If an acceptable healthy wet nurse can be found this will suffice. Under no circumstances should babies be fed cow or goat milk, which was meant for animals. These have such a different constitution as to be unacceptable. If you cannot find human milk for your baby feed it a combination of various grain and seed milks. Do NOT simply feed it soy milk, as this is too limited and the isoflavone content would be too much. Give your baby a variety of soy, rice, oat and almond milks. This will not equal human milk, but will be nutritionally sound and is infinitely better than cow or other animal milk. The fact that two thirds of Americans were weaned on cow milk is frightening, and the results are reflected in our present society that is so far away from following natural laws. Clinical studies comparing breast fed people to those raised on cow milk show better health, higher I.Q., stronger immunity and other benefits in the breast-fed ones.

Since you will only be eating two meals a day life is going to be much simpler. Would you rather not eat breakfast or not eat lunch? Or you can vary this day to day depending on your mood. Since working people often have so little time in the morning and are so hurried, it might be better to eat only lunch and dinner. If you do prefer to eat breakfast make it very light with whole grain cold cereal and non-dairy milk, or hot whole grain cereal, whole grain bread and herbal tea. Soymilk contains about 120 calories per cup, so this isn't necessary as a beverage since this would add over 800 calories a week. Regular tea is full of caffeine and coffee is not part of a healthy lifestyle. It is a good idea to take your own lunch to work every day for a lot of reasons. A good lunch would include brown rice or other grain, a green or yellow vegetable, a thermos of hot soup, fresh salad, or bread. You can learn to make very interesting sandwiches without meat, poultry or dairy. Most offices have facilities for people who bring their lunch and you can eat a much more delicious meal from home than eating in a restaurant. Dinner should be the main meal of the day. A grain should be your principal food of course. A good dinner would not be very different from lunch with a grain or whole wheat pasta, beans, a green or yellow vegetable, some seafood if desired and bread, soup and salad. The idea of dessert is mostly a western one. Temporarily you can fix macrobiotic desserts, but only as a transition. Enjoy a piece of local fruit, especially in warm climates and in summer if you feel the need for something sweet. You will be surprised at how little you can eat and feel completely satisfied. Do not snack between meals or after dinner. Never eat after dinner, as your stomach should be empty when you go to bed.

Some people may ask "why cook our foods?" You'll notice animals do not naturally eat cooked foods, and cooking our food is one thing that has given man freedom and independence. Fire is one of the four primordial elements (earth, wind and water being the other three) and is basic to preparing our food. It seems to escape the advocates of a raw food diet that we're not animals and aren't limited to raw foods. Cooking is necessary for such things as grains and beans. Heat transforms our food and makes it more digestible. When you steam or stir-fry vegetables they keep most all of their nutrition. Cooking is very yang and changes the very nature of our food. If you look at people who have been on a raw food diet for any length of time you'll see they are pale, weak, sickly, have poor immunity and bad skin. Their choice of foods is also very limited. Usually they are sugar addicts and eat a lot of fruit juice, dried fruit, tropical fruit and sweeteners of various kinds. They are far too yin, which you can see reflected in their poor judgment and way of life. Cooking is a divine art, a sacred ceremony and the kitchen is the center of the home. Use the magic of fire to change the very quality of your food.

There are no cookbooks recommended here. The macrobiotic cookbooks are pretty plain, uninteresting and uncreative being based on Japanese culture and not the universal cuisine of the world. Go to your local library and get cookbooks from around the world and use them to create interesting, varied, creative and delicious meals without watering down the health benefits of macrobiotics. Chinese is generally the best and there are five different regional styles to choose from. Often you need make no changes at all in the recipes. Indian food uses too much fenugreek, pepper, cumin, hot chilies, mustard, coconut milk, cardamon, tamarind, cayenne and other stimulating tropical spices for regular meals. Burmese, Mongolian, and Filipino are exotic, different and interesting. Southern Italian cooking uses too much tomatoes and dairy cheese and it is very hard to substitute for tomatoes.

Northern Italian cooking uses too much meat and dairy cheese. Thai cooking uses too many tropical spices like hot chilies, curries (different from Indian curry), serrano peppers and coconut milk for regular use, but these can be omitted. Vietnamese cooking offers many possibilities with only small changes. Korean has potential but is the least healthy of all Asian cooking styles. Cajun cooking has little to offer due to its highly spicy nature and use of animal foods and fats. Eastern European cooking is very meat and dairy oriented and uses many nightshade vegetables. Classical Northern European (English, Welsh, Irish, Scottish, German, Austrian) cooking is a meat and potatoes diet by tradition. When is the last time you saw a Swedish, Finnish, Norwegian, Danish or Swiss restaurant? French country cooking is infinitely better than the high fat classic French and has some real potential. Latin, Central and South

American cooking offers possibilities when whole grains are used and tropical fruits and nightshade vegetables are omitted. Middle Eastern food can be very applicable to whole grain healthy meals. Mexican cooking has a lot going for it when you take the cheese and meat out of it. Unfortunately black Americans cannot look to African cooking for inspiration, as even the Ethiopian is too undeveloped. The healthiest recipes are going to come from China as well as Vietnam. Most people find the various regional Chinese styles to be the most practical and enjoyable especially the stir-fried vegetables. There is a lot you can do with standard American cooking and some imagination to make healthful meals. Japanese cooking is very healthy but very limited, restrictive and uncreative and just not fun. And this one cuisine has been the basis for macrobiotics for no reason at all except the authors were born in Japan. For over 30 years now millions of people have limited themselves to this without questioning it. Use the cuisines of the world to inspire you to eat whole healthy natural food in tune with the universal laws.

Chapter 18: Condiments and Seasonings

Eating should be fun, delicious and most enjoyable. One of the reasons Japanese macrobiotics is understandably not appealing to many people is the severe and very unnecessary restrictions on seasonings, flavors and condiments. The Japanese actually cook very little food and have the most limited and uncreative cooking style in Asia. Eating this way is just not very flavorful, fun and enjoyable. The seasonings seem to be limited to such things as tamari soy sauce, ginger, miso, bonita shavings, natto, and other such Japanese traditions. There is just no reason at all for this. Food should be delicious, flavorful, aesthetic, pleasing and fully seasoned without the use of fats and hot spices using all the healthful international styles available.

The key to using the following seasonings is *moderation*. There are many flavorings that can enhance your food when used with a light hand such as sage, rosemary, basil, thyme, tarragon, oregano, bay leaf, cumin, marjoram, mint, lemon grass, caraway seed, celery seed, good vinegars, horse radish, Italian seasoning, mustard, nutmeg, garlic, coriander leaf and seed, parsley, orange peel, lemon and lime peel, lemon and lime juice (in small amounts). Others include Chinese soy sauce, dry sherry, vanilla, Thai fish sauce, Old Bay seasoning, Worcestershire sauce and capers. Soy cheese can be used in all the regular dairy flavors, soy milk, soy yogurt, soy sour cream and other soy products will replace most any dairy product. Toasted nuts such as walnuts, almonds, filberts and pecans make an elegant garnish especially to stir fried vegetables. It is true we should avoid or limit powerful hot spices such as black pepper, cayenne pepper, chilies, hot sauce, curries and other such tropical spices.

We should not use nut butters like peanut butter except occasionally in small amounts, as the fat content is far too high. Ketchup is another poor choice even natural ketchup since it is tomato based. Barbeque sauce is another tomato-based concoction. Mayonnaise is too full of fat obviously for regular use. Most salad dressings are full of chemicals. The list of these traditional American condiments goes on.

The most important condiment to talk about is salt. We need salt in our diet, although many people will tell you it is somehow harmful to add salt to any food. The Framingham Heart Study proved beyond any doubt that moderate salt use is not harmful and does not contribute to high blood pressure or any other coronary heart condition. Since Americans do eat too much salt and sodium we can understand why many people react to the past and reject the use of salt. We eat so much red meat, cheese and other high sodium foods that we already get an overload of sodium just in the food we eat. In fact salt is very necessary to our lives and should be used in our food. Salt free diets are dull, boring, very unnecessary, and unhealthful if taken too far. The word salt comes from the Latin "sal" and this is what the word "salary" is based on, since Roman soldiers were paid in part with salt.

Salt was one of the most important items of commerce for thousands of years and still is. The Bible is full of references to salt. We've all heard the term, "salt of the earth". Traditional macrobiotics simply used too much salt, however, in such things as miso soup, tamari soy sauce, natto, gomasio (ground sesame seeds and salt), pickled vegetables and pressed salads. You do not need to buy overpriced "sea salt" as all salt comes from the sea; that's right, all salt originated in the oceans and has been deposited on land. Talking about the "importance" of sea salt is scientifically unsound and the minerals this provides are biologically insignificant consisting mostly of very small amounts of magnesium. Simply find a brand that does not use an aluminum anti-caking agent (always avoid anything with aluminum salts in it). Our bodies naturally expel salt in the urine within hours of taking it in, but that is no reason to overdo it. Eating too much salt results in edema (water retention) and unbalances the body, which uses up valuable energy getting rid of the excess water. Use salt intelligently in moderation.

No baking powder or baking soda is used for baking and this is very wise as they are too yin. If you want to bake something occasionally that cannot be leavened with yeast find a sodium based baking powder like Rumford. Never eat anything with aluminum-based baking powder as this is one of the main sources of aluminum in our diets. Aluminum pots are rarely used anymore unless coated with chemically inert Teflon.

Chapter 19:
Calorie Restriction and Fasting

Americans are literally the fattest people on earth and one-third of us are overweight. Obesity is an epidemic that only gets worse every year. What has happened in the last 30 years? What has changed? Look at any movie or television shows filmed around 1970 or earlier and you don't see all these fat people. It would be nice to be able to answer this question since it seems nothing basic has changed in three decades. For example, fast food outlets were popular and the meat, potatoes and sugar diet was as common then as it is now. It is not just that we eat too much, but almost half the calories we eat are fat calories. Most all of the fat calories are saturated animal fats. It isn't the food per se that makes you fat, but the FAT you eat. The rural Red Chinese eat more calories than we do, but much more grains and vegetables and far less fat. Refined grains, empty calories and the 125 pounds of sweeteners we eat every year all add to this. Lack of exercise is certainly a factor, but people were just as lazy thirty years ago. We are the richest nation on earth, have the least expensive food supply, the highest standard of living materially, so we eat the most food per person and the most fat. We're the fattest nation on earth and lead every nation in most any disease rate you can name. Obesity equals disease and short life span.

You can eat as much as you want if you make good food choices. Diets don't work; they never have worked and never will work. Just make better food choices. The answer is making more intelligent, informed and aware, food choices to be in harmony with the universe that created and sustains us. You cannot go hungry for long because the hunger instinct is too deeply imbedded for survival and is much, much stronger than even our sexual instinct. You can go without sex your entire life, but it's hard to go without food for even a day. If you eat whole grains, beans, vegetables, seafood, salads and fruits you can eat all you want and not be overweight. That's right, if you eat whole natural foods you can satisfy your hunger and not gain weight.

The first thing you can do is stop eating three meals a day. You do not need to eat three times a day regardless of the fact 99% of Americans do this. In fact you can eat a snack in the morning like a bowl of hot or cold whole grain cereal and only eat one real meal a day in the evening. Would you rather skip breakfast or lunch? Or you can alter which meal you will skip as you feel like it. Many people will prefer to drop breakfast as they have so little time in the morning to prepare and eat food and are in a hurry to get to work. Drop down to eating two meals a day and stop eating three times a day. The less you eat the better you'll feel, the healthier you will be, the less illness you will get and the longer you'll live. Ben Franklin said, "To lengthen thy life, lessen thy meals".

Eating fewer calories — not necessarily less food- slows the aging process and extends maximum life span. Glucose and insulin metabolism are improved, body temperature is lowered, immunity is enhanced, less illness and less severity of illness occurs as well as less oxidative stress. Calorie restriction does not mean going hungry, but rather eating whole, natural nutrient dense foods that are low in fat and high in fiber and nutrition. This is *not* a matter of eating less food and going hungry at all. More and more scientific evidence comes in every month proving that calorie restriction is the single most powerful and effective means of extending our life span. The less you eat the longer you live. The average active woman only needs about 1,200 calories per day and the average active man only about 1,800 calories. Generally we eat at least twice that here in America and the results are all too obvious.

There has been quite a bit of research on the benefits of calorie restriction especially on animals including monkeys. Of course it would take almost a century to fully do this for humans, but there has been a lot of shorter-term human research as well. The animal studies have shown this works best when started from birth, but has dramatic benefits even when begun in middle or older aged people. Typical of this is a group effort done with real people at the University of Wisconsin, Columbia University and the Veterans Administration (Toxicol. Sci. 1999, v. 52, p. 35-40). People on calorie restriction for just a few years had much better health than the control group and much better prospects for not only living longer but getting less diseases of most every kind.

With all this published research on calorie restriction you would think there would be a good number of books written on this subject as well as magazine articles. Unfortunately this isn't true and there only seems to one author on this subject. Roy Walford wrote "The 120 Year Diet and Maximum Lifespan," which you should read if you have to get your local library to borrow them.

(His third book, sorry to say, is not worth reading as he changed his course quite a bit).

Along with calorie restriction goes fasting. Fasting means water only; there is no other definition. People who speak of "juice fasts" really mean juice feasts. You can fast for a week very easily and this is good enough for most people to do once a year. Very heavy people can fast longer and they can consider a multiple and vitamin supplement for fasts longer than a week. As Christ said 2,000 years ago when his disciples could not heal an afflicted man, "This kind goeth out not, but by prayer and by fasting". The Old and New Testaments are full of references to fasting that are almost always ignored or explained away in modern churches. All religions have a long tradition of fasting especially the Buddhists, Hindus, Moslems and Mormons. Christ fasted for forty days in the desert before beginning his ministry. Buddha fasted and meditated to become enlightened. People who meditate should use fasting to deepen their sessions. You don't have to be a religious person to fast, though, as fasting builds inner strength and character while healing, repairing and cleansing the body and clearing the mind. The wilderness animals know the value of fasting when they are sick or injured. Pythagoras the philosopher required his initiates to undergo a long fast before they could be accepted into his mystery school to prove their character and sincerity.

Fortunately there are some excellent books on fasting. Patricia Bragg's "The Miracle of Fasting", Alan Cott's "Fasting-The Ultimate Diet", Lee Bueno's "Fast Your Way to Health", Dave Williams' "The Miracle Results of Fasting", Herbert Shelton's "Fasting for Renewal of Life", Norbert Kriegisch's "Healthy Fasting", and Eve Adamson's new "Complete Idiot's Guide to Fasting" are all good to read. Once you read some of these books you'll come to see that fasting is *enjoyable* and has great rewards. This is not about deprivation, suffering and being hungry at all.

The simplest and easiest way to start fasting is to choose one day a week to go 24 hours on water only. Do this 52 weeks a year. Every week fast for one whole day, and this will become a most meaningful and enjoyable ritual for you. Eat your dinner and do not eat again until dinner the next day. If a special occasion comes up just fast the day before or the day after, but always honor your weekly one day fast. This will give your body 52 days a year to rest, relax, purify and repair itself. Taking a two-day fast once a month is another good habit to get into. After a while this will become normal to you and the two days will pass very quickly

83

with no side effects at all. Our bodies are self-healing and self-repairing, especially when we go without food for a period of time and only drink water. The 15th century physician Paracelsus said, "Fasting is the greatest remedy- the physician within." There is no more powerful healing method than fasting.

Surprisingly, feelings of hunger usually cease after the third day and, ironically, longer fasts can actually be easier, since there is little desire for food. At first some people may experience mild side effects as toxins and poisons are expelled from their systems. The less side effects you have the healthier you are; the more side effects you experience the more you needed to fast. Headaches and a feeling of general sickness happen temporarily in some people, but these tend to go away quickly. Do not end your fast if you have side effects. Quite the contrary, this shows just how much you need to get these accumulated poisons out of your system. You will actually feel happy, euphoric, clear headed, light and energetic when you don't eat although a little weaker physically.

Pregnant and nursing women should not fast more than one day. Diabetics can learn to fast by healing themselves and going longer and longer periods without food and getting off their insulin. Children and the elderly can certainly fast as can your pets when they are ill.

Chapter 20: Calorie Density of Foods

This is how many pounds of each food a person would have to eat every day in order to get 2,500 calories. For example you could only eat 10 ounces of vegetable oil at one extreme or try to eat more than 25 pounds of zucchini squash. You could eat a 15-ounce bag of almonds or try and finish off over 16 pounds of peaches. The caloric intake would be the same. The grains and beans are cooked in the normal manner. Vegetables, fruits, seafood, poultry and meat are raw. Values do vary here, but not by much.

Vegetable Oil 0.6
Butter 0.8
Almonds 0.9
Peanuts 0.9
Peanut Butter 0.9
Pistachios 0.9
Sesame Seeds 0.9
Walnuts 0.9
Cashews 1.0
Chocolate Candy 1.0
Cheez-Its™ 1.0
Sirloin Steak 1.2
Beef Chuck 1.4
Blue Cheese 1.5
Cream Cheese 1.5
Sugar 1.5
Coconut 1.6
Honey 1.8
French Fries 1.7
Potato Chips 2.0
Tuna (oil) 1.9
Turkey 2.1
Ground Beef 1.9
Corn Chips 2.0
Ham 2.1
Mackerel 2.3
Lamb Chops 2.2
Pork 2.1

WW Pasta 3.1
Chicken 3.2
Avocado 3.3
Eggs (whole) 3.4
Veal 3.4
Chestnuts 3.5
Salmon 3.9
WW rolls 4.0
Tuna (water) 4.3
Chickpeas 4.6
Millet 4.6
Olives 4.7
Navy Beans 4.8
Brown Rice 5.1
Soybeans 4.9
Scallop 4.9
Shrimp 4.8
Pink Beans 5.0
Pinto Beans 5.3
Sweet Potato 5.4
Lentils 5.4
Black Beans 5.5
Kidney Beans 5.6
Lobster 5.8
Crab 5.9
Buckwheat 5.9
Oatmeal 6.0
Yams 6.3

Bananas 6.4
Corn 6.5
Green Peas 6.5
Prunes 6.8
Raspberries 7.5
Tofu 7.6
Mangoes 8.3
Cherries 8.7
Blueberries 8.8
Pears 9.0
Plums 9.1
Nectarines 9.3
Apples 9.4
Blackberries 9.4
Potatoes 9.6
Soymilk 10.1
Pineapple 10.5
Apricots 11.4
Grapes 11.9
Soy Sprouts 11.9
Collards 12.1
Brussels Sprouts 12.1
Cranberries 12.4
Seaweeds 12.4
Beets 12.7
Carrots 13.0
Onions 14.8
Strawberries 14.8
Okra 15.2

Oranges 15.6
Mung Sprouts 15.6
Tangerines 16.1
Peaches 16.6
Pumpkin 16.6
Mustard Greens 17.6
Cantaloupe 18.2
Melons 18.2
Persimmon 19.5
Mushrooms 19.5
Cauliflower 20.2
Asparagus 21.0
Spinach 21.0
Watermelon 21.0
Green Beans 21.9
Cabbage 22.8
Artrichokes 26.0
Endive 27.3
Grapefruit 27.3
Watercress 27.3
Eggplant 28.8
Squash 28.8
Zucchini 32.1
Radish 32.1
Celery 32.8
Cucumbers 32.8
Lettuce 39.0

Meat, dairy, poultry and eggs have the highest calorie density because of their high fat content. Grains and beans are low so you can eat all you want. Fruit are very low in calories, but their high sugar dictates eating in moderation. Green and yellow vegetables generally contain less calories than any other food, and you can eat as many of these as you want; in fact if you ate only green and yellow vegetables you couldn't get enough calories to live.

Chapter 21: Feed Your Pets Well

One third of American families own dogs and cats. Do you really love your pet? Then why are you feeding them that awful commercial pet food; because it is convenient and cheap? Feed them delicious, naturally healthy food they will enjoy. Animals cannot eat the foods we eat because they have a different digestive system and teeth. Our pets have short digestive systems meant for digesting meat and teeth meant to rip and tear flesh; this is their biological nature. Animals usually only eat once a day in the wild and this is also a good idea for domesticated ones. Feed them warmed food, as smell is very crucial to their life. Your dog and cat is meant to eat meat and animal foods and must have them to thrive. Fish and seafood can be a good staple especially for cats. Do not feed your pet milk and dairy foods as, like all the other animals, they do not eat these in their natural state. They are as lactose intolerant as we are. Buddhist monks feed their temple cats a mixture of fish and whole grains like barley and rice as they realize cats cannot exist on the same diet they eat. Misguided vegetarians feed their cats and dogs a pure vegetarian diet, which results in sickness and early death. Animals are meant to eat animal foods and must have at least half of these in their food to be healthy and well.

A good standard is to feed your pet half animal food and half whole grains with some green or yellow vegetables added. It is important to see they get some small amount of green or yellow vegetables for their vitamin A and other needs. They do eat this way in the wild and one reason you'll see them eat grass. Again, do not feed them milk or dairy foods, except for occasional hard cheese, which contain almost no lactose. It is very easy to find inexpensive cuts of pork, beef, chicken, turkey, various organ meats (like liver, kidneys, hearts, brains), fish, shellfish and eggs. Most supermarkets have a section where outdated meat is sold at half price and this is a great way to find inexpensive cuts of good food for your pet. Talk to the butcher about inexpensive types of meat and organs in bulk that can be frozen.

If you knew what was in commercial pet food you would never again feed this to your beloved friends. If you went to a pet food factory and saw the ingredients allowed by law to be put into them you would never buy any again. Diseased animals, for example, are a main ingredient; also a high fat content. Commercial pet foods, no matter how well advertised, are not fit for your pet. It just takes a few minutes a day to feed them what you would want if you were them.

Your pets can also benefit greatly from many of the same supplements you use. Beta glucan, flax oil, acidophilus, beta-sitosterol, multi-vitamins and minerals, glucosamine, L-glutamine, PS, CoQ10, curcumin, quercitin and others can be added to their diet especially as they age and get older and need these. It is important to understand that they should get amounts proportionate to their weight. If you have a 150-pound German Shepard you can give it the same amounts of supplements you take. If you have a 15-pound Pekinese it only needs one-tenth the amount you would need.

It would take a specialist to test the hormone levels of your cat or dog as they get older and most people would not be willing to do this. You can give them melatonin when they get older, but by body weight. If you have had your male dog castrated or your female dog's ovaries removed they have a severe hormone imbalance and an equally severe biological imbalance from such destructive surgery. Yes, it is important to keep unwanted puppies from being born and tying of the seminal vesicles and tubal ligation are much less harmful means of doing this. Would you cut the testicles off your son or cut the ovaries out of your daughter? Aren't your pets like children to you?

Be sure they get a long walk twice a day with you. This is their "hunting time" and you are members of their pack. Walking with you is more than just exercise — it is instinctual and part of the bonding experience with their pack. Good food and exercise will prevent them from gaining weight. Don't share any junk food or sweets, as this is not a real treat at all. If they are sick let them go without food for a day or two as they would in the wild, as fasting is instinctual with them.

Chapter 22: Meditation

How can you call macrobiotics "Zen macrobiotics" without talking about meditation? Do you know what the word "zen" in Japanese means? It simply means meditation just like "chan" does in Chinese. Daily formal meditation should be the spiritual center of your life.

A person who thinks all the time, has nothing to think about but thoughts, and thus becomes disconnected from the direct reality of the world. Reality is neither materialistic, nor spiritual, nor both, nor neither. It is something that cannot be said, written, communicated or described. And if you can't say it, you can't sing it either. As Krishnamurti said, "there are no deep thoughts; all thoughts are shallow." The most difficult of all things is to have a silent mind beyond thought. Nothing is more difficult than this as it is the door to Enlightenment. In meditation you are only concerned with the here and now. "Be here now" may be the best mantra of all. The past is a memory and the future a dream. When the knower becomes one with the known you have reached. An important tenet of Zen is "no purpose". But how does one give up purpose except by having a purpose to give it up? There is only one Universal Ground of being underlying all phenomena. Sat Chit Ananda in Hinduism — consciousness, energy, bliss.

There really are no meditation techniques, as this would clearly imply purposeful behavior. There is something you can do though. Simply watch your breath. No breathing techniques here — just silently watch your breath. You'll see it is neither voluntary nor involuntary. Just quietly watch your breathing and you'll notice it becomes deeper and stronger without any effort at all. Quite the contrary, if you make any efforts it will not happen. An old Zen aphorism is, "If you strive you fail, if you don't strive you fail. What else is there?" After a while you will hardly breath at all while you meditate; just two or three breaths a minute instead of a dozen.

Why should you sit with your back straight up and your legs loosely crossed? It is because this is actually the most comfortable way to sit for prolonged periods. Ideally an hour of meditation a day is enough. This can be divided into half hour morning and half hour evening periods if you want.

If you have never read or heard of Alan Watts, he could be considered the premier American writer on Zen. The main book you should read is "The Book". His other books include: *The Art of Meditation, Meditation, The Wisdom of Insecurity, Nature, Man & Woman, Tao: The Watercourse Way, Nonsense, This Is It, What Is Tao?, Still the Mind, The Supreme Identity, Myself: A Case of Mistaken Identity, Cloud-Hidden, Whereabouts Unknown, Behold the Spirit, Zen and The Beat Way, The Spirit of Zen, Buddhism, Myth & Ritual in Christianity, Two Hands of God, Psychotherapy East & West, What is Zen?, In My Own Way and Does It Matter?* There are also a variety of tapes, videos, books edited after his death by his son and books about Alan himself.

D.T. Suzuki is another excellent author. His books include "Zen Buddhism", "Zen Doctrine of No Mind", and others. Many audio tapes are now available as well. He is one of the finest writers on the Zen tradition ever.

J. Krishnamurti wrote a variety of books. He is not the most entertaining or fun person to read, and comes off as rather serious and his books somewhat dry. What he says in them though will change your life and leave no doubt about his enlightenment. They include: *Meeting Life, Think on These Things, This Light in Oneself, Freedom from the Known, Education and the Significance of Life and The First and Last Freedom. Jiddu is someone who will change your life.*

If you want a real iconoclast read Bhagwan Shree Rajneesh (aka Osho). Instead of listening to the media about him, read one of his books and see for yourself. If there is one thing he emphasizes, it is that life has no meaning at all without meditation, without understanding who and what you are. He is very funny and very unique and criticizes everyone from Mother Theresa and the Pope to Mahatma Gandhi. He wrote dozens of books and many of them are still available, as are the video tapes. You can't take yourself seriously if you want to read "Osho".

Chapter 23: Books to Read

- Dean Ornish: Eat More, Weigh Less
    Program for Reversing Heart Disease
- Anthony Satarillo: Recalled by Life
- Gary Null:
    Get Healthy Now
    Vegetarian Handbook
    Seven Steps to Perfect Heatlh
- Kohler: Healing Miracles from Macrobiotics
- Susan Powter:
    Stop the Insanity
    Food
- Virginia Brown: Macrobiotic Miracle
- John McDougall
    The McDougall Program
    The McDougall Program for a Healthy Heart
    The McDougall Program for Women
- Milenka Dobic: My Beautiful Life
- Elaine Nussbaum: Recovery from Cancer
- Robert Pritikin:
    The New Pritikin Program
    Pritikin Weight Loss Breakthrough
    Pritikin Principle
    Healthy Eating for Life for Women
    Physician's Committee for Responsible Medicine
- Michio Kushi:
    Cancer Prevention Diet
    Macrobiotic Approach to Cancer
    Diet for a Strong Heart
    The Macrobiotic Way
    The Cancer Prevention Diet
    Macrobiotic Diet
    The Book of Macrobiotics
    Standard Macrobiotic Diet
- George Ohsawa:
    You Are All Sanpaku
    Zen Macrobiotics
    Order of the Universe

Macrobiotics- The Art of Healing
Essential Ohsawa
- Dave Williams: Miracle Results of Fasting
- Lee Bueno: Fast Your Way to Health
- Joel Fuhrman: Fasting-and Eating- for Health
- Herbert Shelton: Fasting for Renewal of Life
- Patricia Bragg: Miracle of Fasting
- Eve Adamson: Complete Idiot's Guide to Fasting
- Alan Cott: Fasting - The Ultimate Diet
- Terry Shintani: The Hawaii Diet
- Norbert Kriegisch: Healthy Fasting
- William Dufty: Sugar Blues
- Roy Walford:
  The 120 Year Diet
  Maximum Lifespan
- Bradley Willcox: The Okinawa Program
- Neal Barnard:
  Live Longer, Live Better
  Food for Life
  Eat Right, Live Longer
  Turn off the Fat Genes

OTHER BOOKS FROM NEW CENTURY PUBLISHING 2002

No More Horse Estrogen! - Roger Mason $ 7.95 US
                                                        $11.95 CAN

The Natural Prostate Cure - Roger Mason $ 6.95 US
                                                        $10.95 CAN

What Is Beta Glucan? - Roger Mason $ 4.95 US
                                                        $ 6.95 CAN

Lower Cholesterol Without Drugs - Roger Mason $ 6.95 US
                                                        $10.95 CAN

A Doctor in Your Suitcase $ 9.95 US
                                                        $14.95 CAN

Natural Born Fatburners $14.95 US
                                                        $19.95 CAN

Nutritional Leverage for Great Golf $ 9.95 US
                                                        $14.95 CAN

Cancer Disarmed $ 4.95 US
                                                        $ 6.95 CAN

Kids – First: Health with No Interference $12.95 US
                                                        $19.95 CAN

Overcoming Senior Moments $ 7.95 US
                                                        $11.95 CAN

To order contact:
(413) 229-7935
US (888) NATURE-1

Safe Goods Publishing
561 Shunpike Road
Sheffield, MA 01257